Overcoming Common Problems Series

Selected titles

A full list of titles is available from Sheldon Press,
36 Causton Street, London SW1P 4ST and on our website at
www.sheldonpress.co.uk

Overcoming Common Problems Series

Overcoming Common Problems Series

To Dan, Louis and Max

Family quarrels are bitter things. They don't go according to any rules. They're not like aches or wounds, they're more like splits in the skin that won't heal because there's not enough material.

(F. Scott Fitzgerald)

Contents

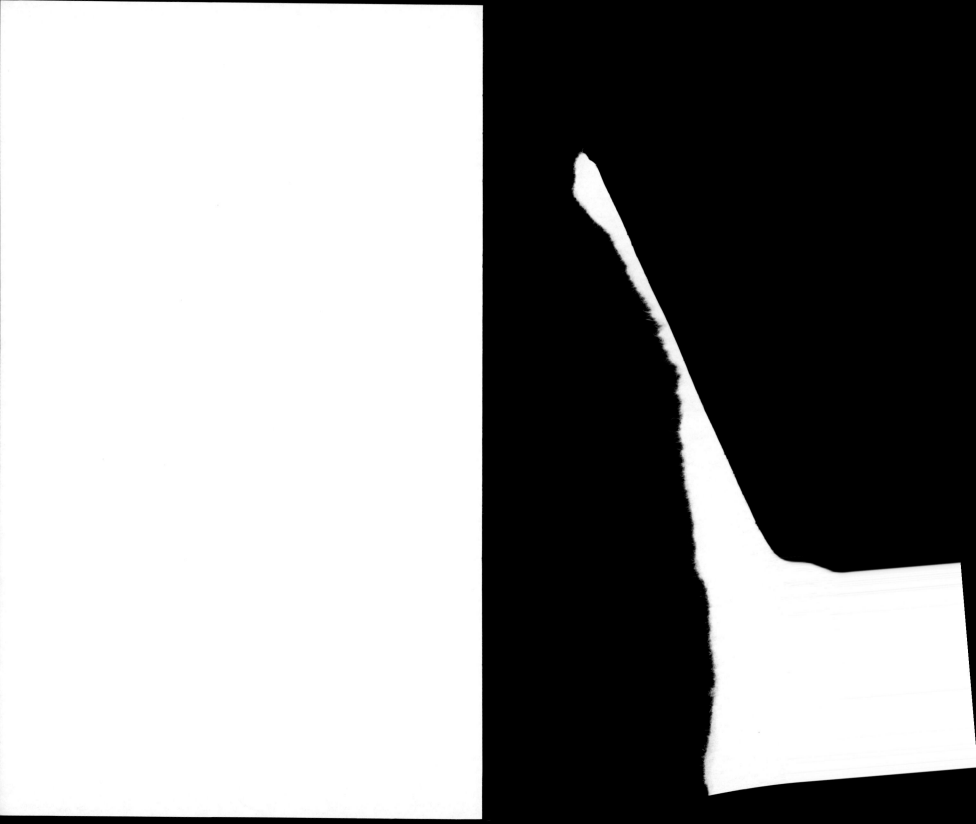

Acknowledgements

This book would not have been possible without the help of many people who gave up their valuable time to talk to me or agreed to let me reproduce the results of their hard work in the field of families and drug addiction. In no particular order, I would like to thank: Dr Nicky Rycroft of London South Bank University for helping with the science and giving me her insights into the nature of addiction; Bernie Oldbury of Solihull Integrated Addiction Services, who very kindly allowed me to draw on the excellent supporting material for their Family and Friends Information Programme; Sam Smithers of Grandparents Plus and Grant Reyland of the Grandparents Association for their insights into grandparent and kinship caring; Professor Anthony Jorm of the University of Melbourne for permission to reproduce guidelines on dealing with aggression; Professor Richard Velleman, Dr Lorna Templeton, Professor Jim Orford and Professor Alex Copello for allowing me to draw on their extensive work in this field, both individually and as the UK Alcohol Drugs and the Family Research Group; Professor Marina Barnard for permission to quote from her highly insightful book, *Drug Addiction and Families*; Rebecca Linssen and Dr George Sanju for generously sharing their contacts; Oliver French at Adfam for invaluable help with contacts and case studies; Jane Brown, projects manager at the West Sussex Drug and Alcohol Action Team, for her insights into the workings of support groups; the helpful and knowledgeable staff of the British Library in general and Jeremy in the Science Room in particular, who spent a great deal of time and effort helping me track down studies; and Cathy Ashley of the Family Rights Group for helping me access families who have suffered from a member's drug use. It goes without saying that any errors and omissions are entirely mine.

The family members who gave up their time to talk to me about painful and personal events and feelings deserve a special category of thanks. They were willing to share their stories with a total stran-

names and identifying details but I hope that I have managed to preserve their voices and their experiences. I thank them from the bottom of my heart.

Finally, I would like to thank my own family – my husband Dan and my two sons Louis and Max. This book is dedicated to them and would not have been possible without their love, support and willingness to let me disappear for entire weekends in order to write.

Introduction

If you're reading this book, chances are that you are concerned about someone close to you who is a drug user. It might be your mother, your father, your cousin, your brother, your son or even a friend. Whoever you are concerned about, I hope that this book helps and supports you as you decide how to cope with this situation.

First, let me reassure you that you are not alone. The drug information charity DrugScope estimates that around 30 per cent of the general adult population have tried an illegal drug. Out of those, it's believed that around 400,000 people in the UK are addicted to heroin and crack. However, it's not known how many people are addicted to other drugs, such as cannabis, ecstasy or ketamine, and the real number of people who are addicted to a drug may be much higher. Each one of these drug addicts has a mother, a sister, a brother or a child who will be affected by the problems that arise from their drug use. A review of the available literature by Richard Velleman and Lorna Templeton in 2007, published in the journal *Advances in Psychiatric Treatment*, estimated that about eight million family members – partners, children, parents, brothers and sisters, or wider family members such as aunts or cousins who take on the caring role – are 'living with the negative consequences of someone else's drug or alcohol misuse' (all details of works referred to are in the 'References' section at the end of the book).

However, although many services exist to help the drug abuser, there are far fewer around to help their families. Support group provision is patchy. Local charities do their best with ever-limited resources. And while there is plenty of research on addiction, far less attention has been paid to the effect an addict's behaviour has on the people who, as several of the family members of drug users that I spoke to for this book put it, 'pick up the pieces' – even though, as research is starting to show, families can have a positive effect on the drug user, and can be a major influence in his or her decision to seek treatment. But leaving aside the question of how best to help the drug user, there is also the undoubted fact that these families need help, however they choose to deal with the user in their midst. We know that having a drug addict in the family can lead to horrific consequences for family members. So more involvement for families would have a doubly positive effect – it would provide help and encouragement for those who wish to work with the drug user in seeking and going through treatment, and it would also provide psychological and actual support for those who don't. As Professor Marina Barnard, who has worked extensively with drug users and their families, points out in her book *Drug Addiction and Families*:

> Problem drug use hits families like a tidal wave, leaving those involved floundering in a sea of anger, frustration, fear and isolation. Yet for all the enormity of this event, it has largely escaped notice. Drugs policy, drug research and service provision has been predominantly about meeting the needs of the individual with the drug problem.   (p. 11)

It's easy to assume, if you've never had contact with drug abuse before, that it's something that happens to the 'bad lads' or lasses, a problem confined to tower blocks and run-down council estates rather than suburbs or country villages. But this is not necessarily the case. While it's certainly true that deprived areas of the UK suffer more than their fair share of drug addiction, it's something that happens in all sections of society, to all walks of life. A DrugScope survey referred to above also asked respondents about social class and found similar levels across the board: 18 per cent of those whose lives had been affected by drug addiction were defined as 'AB' – the professional, moneyed class; 20 per cent were in C1 – defined as lower middle class; and 14 per cent were in C2, the skilled working class.

> The first year of his addiction that we knew of, I didn't believe that he was 'a drug addict'. I thought no, he's not like that. You always imagine drug addicts to be lying in the gutters, dirty – Steve was this clean boy, clean clothes every day, shower or bath twice a day. It took a long time for it to actually get home to me that, yes, he was an addict.
>
> (Miriam, mother of heroin addict Steve)

We were from a 'nice' family. We had money, a nice house, we'd been to good schools. We'd wanted for nothing. We had happy childhoods and supportive parents. Why did Ben become a heroin addict? I don't really know.   (Marcus)

Whether it's your son, husband, daughter or mother, having a problematic drug user in the family is disastrous. It raises questions that you are unlikely to ever have considered before. Should you continue to allow a drug user to live with you? What should you do if he or she steals from you? What's the best way to encourage him or her to seek treatment? Can you help him or her 'detox' by yourself? What are the health risks to the addict and the family? Why has he or she become addicted in the first place? If the drug addict is a parent, what will happen to the children? And, most importantly, what help is available to help your family get through this?

Those I have spoken to for this book have talked of the 'cycle', the 'merry-go-round' and the 'rollercoaster' of having a drug addict in the family. It is certainly a long, painful journey, to use yet another metaphor. This book does not provide any easy answers. I wish it could. But dealing with a drug addict in the family, sadly, does not slot neatly into the medical model of symptoms, diagnosis, treatment, cure.

I have drawn heavily on research, published in peer-reviewed journals, in an attempt to draw together current thinking on families and drug abuse in a way that's helpful to families. But this, of course, has a danger: real-life situations rarely mirror the relatively controlled nature of scientific research – something every psychologist, psychiatrist and sociologist would agree with. Every drug addict is different, every family is different and every family situation is different. Therefore, how you choose to deal with your situation is intensely personal to you. There are no right or wrong answers. There are different schools of thought, certainly, but there is no single guaranteed way.

Research shows that the families of drug addicts want two things. First, they want help for themselves. They recognize the effect that the drug user is having on their family and they want to take steps to combat that effect. They want advice, information, a listening ear and to hear the experiences of others. Second, they want to know how they can help the drug user. This help may take the form of finding appropriate treatment.

I hope this book will help to fulfil those needs. You will find information on exactly what addiction is, how it is defined and who becomes an addict. You will find a rundown on the major drugs of addiction and their symptoms. You will find suggestions on coping with your own feelings and helping other family members to cope, suggestions for helping the addict to help him or herself – should you choose to do so – and information on the practical support available.

Throughout the book, I have also included the voices of those I have spoken to who have experienced the disruption and misery of having an addict in their own family. Drug abuse in the family is something that many people (understandably) feel unable to talk about and I am extremely grateful to them for sharing these intensely personal and upsetting experiences and feelings.

Drug addiction is a hugely controversial subject and differing opinions arouse very strong feelings. The debates over, for example, the 'war on drugs', legislation and prohibition, harm reduction and heroin on prescription have already filled many books. However, these are subjects for other books. What I'm concerned with is offering support to those whose lives have been affected by drugs and avoiding the political hot potatoes which, although they affect the wider view, are not really relevant to those who simply want help, now. This book is written from, as far as possible, an apolitical stance which does not seek to judge. It simply seeks to offer a helping hand to those who have been affected by a drug addict close to them.

No family member should be left to deal with such a problem alone. If you have bought this book, then you have taken the first step towards seeking help and support. I hope you find it useful.

A word about language

It's worth noting that many health professionals prefer not to use the word 'addict' as it's a very loaded and, for some, derogatory term. For some, it implies the stereotypical heroin addict crouching in a filthy flat – and while this does happen, the reality of substance misuse can be very different depending on the substance and on the person. For others, 'addict' implies a disease over which the sufferer has no control, while others see an addiction as a matter of personal choice which can be overcome by force of will. So you will no doubt encounter many ways of describing what you understand as drugs, addiction and addicts – junkies, substance misuse, substance-use disorder, drug abuse, smackheads, crackheads, stoners, drugs of addiction, harmful use and dependence syndrome.

The debate over exactly what addiction is and what causes it rages on and is unlikely to be resolved soon, if ever. So for the purposes of this book, I will refer to 'addicts' and 'addiction' because these are the terms that the majority of lay people use, and this book is being written primarily with ordinary people, not health professionals, in mind. When discussing the different members of the family, I will also refer to the 'user' – that is to say, the drug user – and the 'carer' – that is, the concerned family member or members. 'Drugs' in this sense also covers use of legal but controlled substances such as aerosols or glue, which are some of the most commonly abused substances in the UK and are certainly responsible for many deaths. (Chapter 6 gives a brief overview of these substances, their street prices and their effects.)

I have also used 'he' in the book when referring to the user, purely for convenience. More men appear to be dependent drug users than women – in 2007 it was estimated that 4.5 per cent of men and 2.3 per cent of women in England are dependent on drugs. More men than women enter treatment, and more men than women are admitted to hospital with drug-related mental health and behavioural disorders. However, addiction knows no gender boundaries and there are many female addicts.

1

What is drug addiction?

'Addiction' has become something of an over-used word. Hundreds of consumer surveys, puff pieces, and press releases rely on its shock value to convince us that we're 'addicted' to everything from Facebook to crisps, from celebrity gossip to expensive car stereos. As a result, that shock value has been considerably diluted, and it is hard for someone who hasn't been through it to appreciate the sheer disruption, heartbreak and misery that an addiction to drugs can cause, both to the user and to his family and social network. Everyone knows the standard media depiction of a drug addict – usually a pimply young man on a council estate – but far fewer recognize the truth: that anyone, from any social class, of any race, gender or age, can become a drug addict.

There are many theories of addiction – what makes an addict? Are some people more likely to become addicts than others? Is addiction a 'disease' or is it a 'choice'? You probably won't be surprised to hear that nobody has yet come up with a definitive answer to all these questions, probably because there isn't one, but in this chapter I aim to give a brief, non-academic overview of current thinking, in order to help you understand a little more about this condition which has come into your family.

The dictionary defines 'addiction' as 'the state of being enslaved to a habit or practice or to something that is psychologically or physically habit-forming, such as narcotics, to an extent that its cessation causes severe trauma'. So when we talk about 'addiction' in this book, we'll be referring to something that's got to the stage of drastically affecting someone's life.

A brief history of addiction

Addiction is not a new problem. The substances may have changed but the problem has always been with us. Alcohol, of course, has been around since humankind first discovered how to ferment grain. There's some evidence to suggest that prehistoric peoples used fungi and other herbs. Cannabis use, it's believed, began in ancient China. Cocaine has been widely used for centuries by South Americans, who chewed the leaves of the coca plant from which the drug derives. The Greek poet Homer, who lived in the ninth century BC, mentions opium, and an Egyptian papyrus has been found, dating from 1500 BC, which mentions the drug. Used initially as a medicine, opium later became the poet's drug of choice, the best-known example being Samuel Taylor Coleridge. Laudanum, a solution of opium, was widely available in the UK and USA in the nineteenth century, and was used both as a medicine to cure ailments such as diarrhoea and to relieve pain, and as a recreational drug. Cocaine was also available from pharmacists during that era – one famous user being Sherlock Holmes, who injected the drug despite admonitions from Dr Watson.

> Count the cost! Your brain may, as you say, be roused and excited, but it is a pathological and morbid process, which involves increased tissue change, and may at least leave a permanent weakness. You know, too, what a black reaction comes upon you. Surely the game is hardly worth the candle. Why should you, for a mere passing pleasure, risk the loss of those great powers with which you have been endowed? (Conan Doyle 1993, p. 89)

(It's interesting to note that Sir Arthur Conan Doyle, Holmes' creator, saw the effects of addiction first-hand in his own family – his father was an alcoholic.)

Gradually, the authorities realized the potential and actual harm of such drugs being available over the counter. In 1916, the UK passed the Defence of the Realm Act, which brought the sale, possession and distribution of cocaine and opium under the control of the Home Office. In 1920, the Dangerous Drugs Act added cannabis and codeine, a derivative of opium, to the list. The government continues to ban new drugs as they emerge and is now even attempting to ban ones which have not yet been manufactured.

However, the problem of addiction and the harm it brings did not go away. New drugs have continued to appear – among them ketamine, ecstasy, LSD, PCP ('angel dust'), crack and, most recently, so-called 'designer drugs' such as mephedrone. Along with the new drugs come new problems and new addicts. The amount of harm done depends on just how addictive the new drug is. Crack, a form of cocaine which can be smoked, ripped through the inner cities of the USA causing harm which is almost impossible to quantify. Intensely addictive and cheap, it ruined thousands of lives, not just through the physical effects of the drug itself but also through the consequences of the addicts' need to get the money for the drug through crime, and the violence caused as rival gangs fought gun battles on the streets for control of lucrative selling spots.

The UK now has the highest levels of addiction and multi-drug consumption and the second-highest rate of drug-related deaths in Europe, according to a report published in 2007 on behalf of the UK Drug Policy Commission. A DrugScope survey of more than 1,000 adults found that a fifth had 'personal experience' of drug addiction. Either they had been or were addicted themselves, or they knew someone who was. Two per cent had experienced drug addiction. Extrapolating from the sample, that's about 1.2 million adults in the UK.

Is your family member an addict?

The Diagnostic and Statistical Manual of Mental Disorders (DSM) is the standard classification of mental disorders used by mental health professionals in the USA and all over the world; it is produced by the American Psychiatric Association. At the time of writing the DSM is currently being revised for the fifth edition.

The new proposed definition which concerns us is 'substance-use disorder'. This is defined as 'a maladaptive pattern of substance use leading to clinically significant impairment or distress' which might manifest itself in many ways. The proposed revisions for DSM 5 state that two or more of the following events occurring over a 12-month period indicate substance-use disorder:

- The sufferer may be repeatedly absent from school or home because of his substance use. He may neglect his home or his family. He may drive a car under the influence of drugs, and continue to use them despite knowing that this use causes tension, arguments or fights. He may stop doing things that he previously enjoyed, like sports or other hobbies.
- In medical terms, he may show a tolerance and need to have more and more of the substance for it to have any effect. If he doesn't get the substance, he'll show withdrawal symptoms.
- The substance may seem to take over his life. He may crave it. He may spend most of his time finding money to buy it, finding a dealer to sell it to him, taking it, recovering from its effects, then having to find money to buy it and starting the cycle all over again.
- He may realize the effect the substance is having and attempt to cut down on it, usually unsuccessfully.
- And he may continue to use the substance even if he knows it's causing him physical and psychological harm.

We know that not everyone who takes drugs is an addict, and there are many people who can use drugs recreationally without becoming addicted. According to DrugScope, 'surveys on a national and local level have found that illegal drug use is only an occasional activity for most people'. The stigma of being an occasional drug user, as opposed to being a drug addict, has also diminished. A study published in the journal *Sociology* in 2002 concluded that recreational drug use, particularly among young people, is becoming increasingly 'normalized', even among those who don't use drugs. Two-thirds of the 465 young adults surveyed who didn't even use drugs still held 'tolerant' or 'approving' views towards drug takers. So it's important to remember that just the act of using drugs does not mean that a person is addicted – though of course the risk is always there and it's far more likely that someone who abuses a drug and isn't yet addicted will become an addict.

Physical and psychological addiction

If you've ever tried to give up smoking, you'll know that there's more to that very common addiction than simply the physical effects of nicotine. You'll probably have found that once the withdrawal symptoms of the drug wear off – irritability, headaches, sleeplessness – you find yourself craving it for other reasons. Perhaps your cigarette was your 'reward' at the end of a hard day, or you felt it helped you concentrate on a difficult piece of work. Perhaps you enjoyed going outside with your workmates for a cigarette break and a gossip. You may not have the physical need for nicotine, but you certainly have a psychological need for the comfort a cigarette gave you.

Drug addiction is similar. Unlike addictions such as gambling, using a drug means that the user's body builds up a tolerance, meaning that he has to take more and more in order to get the desired effect. This leads to actual changes in the brain and body. Take one of the most notorious addictive substances – heroin, or its chemical name, diacetylmorphine. Once it enters the body, it binds to the brain's μ-opioid receptors. This action produces the euphoric effects of the drug – the physical effects. It feels good, so the user takes it again. But the more the user takes it, the more the number of these receptors decreases. The body changes. The user needs to take more to get an effect. If the user stops taking heroin, then those changes will produce the unpleasant physical withdrawal effects known as 'cold turkey' or 'clucking'. So it's easy to see how addiction to heroin can be physical and how a user would take more and more just to stave off the unpleasant withdrawal effects.

But, as with cigarettes, dealing with a heroin addiction isn't just a matter of treating the withdrawal symptoms in the short term and perceiving the addict as cured. There are many more factors affecting drug use which need to be tackled. A study of 107 former problematic drug users asked how they'd managed to kick the habit. Interestingly, few mentioned actual medical treatment. Rather, they spoke of being 'tired of the lifestyle' and consequently taking practical measures like moving away from their drug-using circles, of the support of friends who didn't use drugs, and of religious or spiritual reasons. We know that drug abusers have their own culture, their own rituals, their own language – these can all give a sense of belonging and a very real sense of loss if the user gives up. So there's much more to an addiction than the effect it has on an addict's body, and this extra dimension explains why it's such a difficult thing to recover from. Recovery means turning your back not just on the drug but also on everything that surrounds it – the friends, the good feelings and, in some cases, the only way of adult living that an addict has known. I have used the example of heroin addiction here, as it's one of the most common addictive drugs. But the same applies to any drug.

> I couldn't recall how many counsellors he's seen, how many courses he's been on, how many tests he'd had, that sort of thing. He was on drug testing orders by the court but he knew how to con them and did it, very successfully, so that was a complete waste of time. When he was in prison they gave him advice, courses. He's taken Subutex, methadone, all the substitutes. But he's still gone back on to the heroin.
>
> (Alan, parent of drug addict David)

Why has my family member become addicted?

What drives some people to become addicted to drugs? Why can some people use drugs without becoming addicted? Why do some people choose to try the drugs in the first place, and not others? You'll probably already know the answers to these questions, which is that nobody really knows, though there is no shortage of theories.

You may have asked yourself if it is somehow your fault if a family member has become addicted to drugs. Again, every situation is different. The reasons that people become addicts are as varied as the people themselves. Addiction is a hugely complex disorder which results from many different interplaying factors. So it's highly unlikely that your family member has become an addict as a direct consequence of something you did.

You may be worried that others will judge you. The National

Treatment Agency for Substance Misuse (NTA) noted in its 2008 report, *Supporting and Involving Carers*, that:

> . . . there is a division in the literature between those who consider drug misuse 'a problem *for* the family' and those who consider it 'a problem *of* the family'. Historically, the latter viewpoint has prevailed, with many 'family-blaming' ideas being put forward, which in one way or another stated, 'people develop drug problems because of their parents/spouse'. Taking this approach often means that family members or carers feel stigmatised and unwelcome in treatment settings, and are therefore less likely to seek professional help. Professionals who hold these views are also less likely to invite family members to participate in the misuser's treatment.

But the report goes on to state that:

> More recently, a family-coping framework has started to be developed . . . which suggests that 'people develop drug problems for a wide variety of reasons, and carers/family members have to try to cope with the effects and impact of this on their lives as best as they can'.

This latter approach has been adopted by the many family support services, who will not seek to blame or judge you but will simply help you to cope.

There's a fascinating body of literature, mostly from the 1950s to the 1970s, around women married to alcoholics. Many of these studies saw the wives as having the problem. Wives of alcoholics were stigmatized, described variously as dominating, weak, masochistic or martyrs, with personality disorders bordering on the psychopathic. There was even a theory that men drank because their wives were too 'masculine' – that is to say, they were high-achieving women. Thankfully, things have now moved on and these studies are no longer seen to be relevant. Rather, much research is now focusing on how best a family can help an addict, and how best a family can deal with the chaos an addict brings, rather than seeking to blame the family in the first place.

I don't blame ourselves. The first time we found out he was addicted we thought, dear God, where did we go wrong? But I had two other sons who left school, worked hard, and Steve, who was three years younger than the middle son, he went the opposite way. It did help to know that it wasn't anything we'd done.   (Miriam)

I know that my mother blames herself and I have told her many times that it wasn't her fault – me and him were brought up the same way. We just have different personalities, that's all. You can't blame yourself if your kids have different personalities – that's normal.   (Marcus)

You blame yourself, of course. As parents. You think, what have you done wrong? Not realizing that it's mostly peer pressure. Within our community, in the last eight years, there's been at least five lads of David's age group buried. You'd think that they'd learn from it. But they just think it happened to him, it can't happen to me. We found out that his partner was also an addict. There's some debate over who introduced who to it – I suppose we'll never find out. We're quite open about it now. We don't try and hide it any more. We did at one stage. It did feel shameful but now I'm open about it. It wasn't my doing. We have done everything and more within our power to try and rectify the situation but it is totally out of our control. If he doesn't want to help himself, can we be blamed? I think not.   (Alan)

Genetic predisposition

Genetic predisposition may well be a factor. In short, if you have a history of addiction in the family, you may be more at risk of addiction yourself. But, as ever, it's not as simple as saying that someone's genes have made him the way he is, and there is no single 'addict' gene or personality type which means a person is destined for a lifetime of addiction. Rather, the genetic theory says that genetic influence on addiction comes from whether or not you have a combination of various genes which, in turn, affects how susceptible you are to certain behaviours – for example, one person may have a combination of genes which makes him more susceptible to cocaine use, while another may have a combination which makes him more susceptible to alcohol abuse. It's estimated that genetics and combined genetic–environmental interactions are responsible for around 40 to 60 per cent of the 'variability of risk' of addiction. But, of course, drug addiction doesn't happen in a vacuum. In order to carry out these behaviours, you have to be exposed to the drug in the first place. That's where all the other factors come in.

Environmental factors

These play a vital role in whether or not someone becomes an addict. It stands to reason that if drug abuse is rife in a community, a person is more likely to be exposed to it and therefore more likely to become addicted – it's very hard to resist if all your friends are using and there's a dealer down every street. If drug abuse happens in the family home – for example, if a child has a drug-addicted parent – then the likelihood of that child becoming a drug addict is much stronger. (Though, equally, research shows that it may have the opposite effect and put children off using any drugs as a result of the harm they've seen drugs do to their parents, showing that nothing is ever simple when it comes to theories of addiction.)

Is 'peer pressure' to blame? This is now more generally referred to as 'normalization' – taking into account that peer pressure doesn't happen in a vacuum, either, but against a background where drugs might be more prevalent or where the taking of them is seen as more 'normal'. But the influence of those around you certainly has an effect – although the effect it has will also in turn depend on your state of mental health, your family background and your personality. For example, a US study found that peer pressure to take drugs was more likely to have an effect on teens who didn't live with a father or a stepfather.

Developmental factors

Developmental factors may also be an issue among adolescents. It's now known that certain parts of the brain which regulate our emotions and our ability to judge situations develop later, meaning that teenagers are therefore more susceptible to risky behaviour, and this of course may include using drugs.

The drug of choice

What he chooses to take may also influence whether or not someone becomes addicted, as some drugs are simply more addictive than others. Heroin and cocaine are commonly cited as the most addictive of the illegal drugs, taking into account factors including the pleasure each drug induces and the degree of psychological and physical addiction that they produce.

The gateway theory

This is commonly cited as a pathway to addiction. It runs thus: the person starts off using 'soft' drugs such as cannabis, then progresses to 'harder' drugs such as cocaine and heroin. How does the gateway theory work? Some believe that it's an environmental effect – if you are buying cannabis and smoking it, you're more likely to come into contact with people who are selling or using harder drugs, and therefore you are more likely to be tempted into trying them. Others believe that cannabis, for example, may somehow 'prime' the brain into wanting more substances. Although some studies have found that there seems to be a correlation between soft and hard drug use, others have found no correlation.

Self-medication

Self-medication could be a reason why some people become addicted, particularly in cases where people have physical or psychological disorders that are not being treated at all, or haven't been properly diagnosed, or where the treatment is not having the desired effect. Probably the most well-known example of self-medicating is sufferers of multiple sclerosis using cannabis to treat their symptoms. A person may also self-medicate following a traumatic event if he is suffering from post-traumatic stress disorder (PTSD) – a phenomenon not unknown among military personnel returning from the front line. A Canadian study found that a fifth of PTSD sufferers were self-medicating with drugs or alcohol. Self-medication for psychological disorders is common. Another study published in the *Journal of Affective Disorders* looked at more than 43,000 sufferers of mood disorders including depression and bipolar disorders. Almost a quarter used alcohol or drugs to relieve their symptoms. Having a mental disorder does seem to be a major risk factor for addiction, though this of course begs the question of whether or not drug abuse is common among those who are mentally ill, or whether drug abusers have a high proportion of mental illness.

I think she [Karen] started to have problems from the age of seven. My aunt [Karen's mother] died of cancer and it was quite a slow, lingering death. She [Karen] was aware of it. My aunt wasn't the greatest person at sharing her feelings anyway. She preferred the company of animals. We always did wonder why she ever had children because she didn't seem to be interested in them very much. Karen was born one of twins; her sister died when she was a month old. That cast a big cloud over the family and the way she was brought up. Everyone was always aware that there was one missing. She didn't really have much of a good start in life the way me or my brother did. When she was around seven she started to shut down from everybody. She was difficult to love. You'd give her something like a present and she showed no real emotion. She never showed any emotion to anybody that way. (Carly)

2

How drug addiction
affects the family

When a family member is a drug addict, everyone in that family can become a victim. It may seem obvious to state that drug addiction damages families. But it's worth stating, simply because, while you're caught up in the cycle of having a drug user close to you, it can be hard to stop, sit back and reflect on how the addict's behaviour is affecting you all – not just the addict. The emotional and physical pressure on you and your family is immense and can have serious consequences for your health.

It's easy to focus all your attention on the addict, and sometimes it's not even a conscious choice – you have to get him help, you have to sort out his debts, you have to get him down to the needle exchange. But amid the whirlwind, it is worth weighing up what this behaviour is doing to you, and to your wider family circle, as this may be a factor in any decisions you make about dealing with the addict in the family. As I stated in the introduction, you may have found that there are plenty of services out there focused on helping the drug addict, but not so many which also take into account your needs and those of your family. You may not have been signposted to any family support services in the same way that a drug addict will be signposted towards help.

Again, I'll emphasize that every situation is different and there is no single 'right' way to respond to the revelation that a family member is a drug addict. Don't beat yourself up for reacting the way you did and don't regret actions you may have taken – or actions that you didn't. In such a situation, everyone is groping in the dark and simply trying to get through the best way they can.

The UK Drug Policy Commission report, *Adult family members and carers of dependent drug users: Prevalence, social cost, resource savings and treatment responses*, says:

As well as experiencing harm and much stigma, families of drug users – as is the case in other fields such as mental health and disability – are frequently an unpaid and unconsidered resource providing economic and other forms of support to their drug using relatives and carrying a large burden in terms of costs, which are often to some extent forced upon them. As mentioned, it is widely recognised that a person with an illegal drug problem can have a significant impact on their family members in terms of physical and psychological stress and that those stresses can be severe and long lasting.   (Copello *et al.* 2009)

The report also cites

concern about the drug user's state of physical and mental health as well as his or her behaviour, the reduction of social life for the family and the negative impact on communication between family members. The feelings often associated with these experiences include anxiety, worry, depression, helplessness, anger and guilt.

No doubt these worries will be familiar to you.

Finding out

You may have suspected for a while that something wasn't quite right, and now you know. Perhaps the addict told you himself, or perhaps you confronted him about your suspicions. Perhaps another family member or friend dropped a hint. Either way, it's a shattering shock and its effects should not be underestimated.

We first found out about it when the police knocked on the door. He'd been stopped and was in possession of heroin. Which obviously gave us a shock. He'd agreed to go on a rehab thing, and that meant he must have been a user for a couple of years. I didn't see any signs initially. It was some time before we found out – probably a couple of years. We thought perhaps that he was drinking too much or whatever. Or he'd go away for a few days, presumably to stay with pals.   (Alan)

He said: 'I've been using heroin for two years.' And I knew nothing much about it then. But little things clicked into place. When he was coming in at night he'd be dopey looking and I'd say: 'What have you been doing?' 'Oh, I've had a couple of cans of beer with my friends.' Because I wasn't drug aware, you know, he got told off but you think, well, that's boys growing up. And then another thing was I realized a lot of my spoons were missing. I thought the boys were taking them to work – for yogurts and stuff – even though they all denied it. Little things like that.

(Miriam)

No one ever mentioned it. My nan, my uncle, they never told my mum or myself, or we would have helped. Everyone was so ashamed of what was happening. I think it's a generational thing, especially for my nan. She was so deeply ashamed. She said that she never would have thought that she would ever have a grandchild that took heroin. They were all very worried about Karen. I actually faced them with it and I said: 'You do realize Karen's on drugs, don't you? A child is not born withdrawing from heroin and methadone if the mother's not taking it.' At first they called me a liar. They said: 'Don't be ridiculous.' I said: 'Open your eyes.'

(Carly, cousin of drug addict Karen)

Your first reaction may well be rage: the addict isn't just engaging in self-destructive behaviour, it's also illegal self-destructive behaviour which, if it's being carried out in your house, puts the whole family at risk. We all have hopes for people. We all want those close to us to be happy, to be successful in whatever they choose to do. Now, at a stroke, those hopes have been dashed.

When the initial rage has subsided, you may well enter a period of something very like mourning. Your family member is not the person you thought he was. You've lost that image and you're not sure if you'll ever get him back. Something – trust? hopes? future plans? – has been lost for ever. It is hard to square the happy child in the family album with the sobbing addict who begged forgiveness for stealing your purse. It's hard to adjust your hopes for the future from a wife and child to simply getting him off the drugs.

You might turn to distraction and displacement activities. One way of coping is to throw yourself into practical details. You might spend hours on the internet searching for treatment programmes, support groups, medical treatments, hypnotism – anything that might cure your family member and turn him back into the person you once knew.

Everyday impact

A study by Richard Velleman and Lorna Templeton, 'Understanding and modifying the impact of parents' substance abuse on children', published in the journal *Advances in Psychiatric Treatment* in 2007, identified the following ways in which family life is disrupted by alcohol or drug misuse. Although you may have never encountered some of these disruptions, it's worth reading down the list and thinking about how they might affect your family if they occur in the future.

- Rituals: the ways families celebrate religious or family occasions such as Christmas or birthdays.
- Roles: as one family member develops a substance problem, others take over that person's roles, such as coping with finances, disciplining, shopping and cleaning.
- Routines: when behaviour becomes unpredictable it creates difficulties for the family in planning or committing to routines: will she remember to collect her son from school? When will he come home, and in what state?
- Communication: alcohol and drugs have a major effect on communication between family members.
- Social life: families tend to become increasingly socially isolated, owing to the difficulty of explaining to friends and neighbours that a family member has a drug or alcohol problem, or the social embarrassment or unpredictability associated with drinking and drugs.
- Finances: a family's finances can be hugely affected by reduction in income (owing to job loss, for example) and spending of such income as is obtained on alcohol or drugs instead of more vital items.
- Relationships and interactions: for example, both the misuser and his partner may become much more neglectful of other family members; aggression and violence are much more likely.

How different family members might react

A drug user in the family can affect different members in different ways, depending on many factors – the age of the family member, whether or not he is living at home, his role within the family and, of course, his own personality. The following is just a guide to how the situation might affect each member:

If you're a *parent*, you may be more shocked to discover that your child is using drugs. Drug users can be very good at concealing their activities from parents. It may be more likely, as well, that you have not used drugs or come into contact with those who do. You may also be more likely to take on the caring role, to be the person who researches the treatments, sorts out the sharps box and drags the user down to the doctor. You are also likely to be the person who has to deal with demands for money, or the person who is stolen from.

Siblings can have a different range of reactions. They may take on a protective role, trying to conceal their brother or sister's drug use so that parents don't find out. They may feel angry and resentful towards the drug user and the amount of attention that he is getting from parents. It could also be that they are using drugs as well, and may start using drugs because their sibling is doing so.

Fathers may be less likely to seek support and are more likely to cut themselves off from the drug user as a way of coping. They are less likely to talk about the problem.

Children of drug-using parents are at very serious risk. They are more likely to witness high levels of violence and/or abuse, or to become victims of that abuse themselves. They have a higher risk of developing behavioural and emotional problems, and of being born with physical problems resulting from a parent's drug use in pregnancy. They may also be at physical risk if the drug-taking parent is behaving in dangerous ways – for example, leaving the child alone in the house for long periods, or leaving drugs and injecting equipment around the house. They are also more likely to have to become the carer for a drug-using parent – cooking, cleaning, looking after younger siblings and 'looking after' the drug-using parent if he is suffering withdrawal symptoms or the effects of an overdose. Their education will suffer and they may become socially isolated, unable to bring friends home or go out with friends. (However, it's also known that not all children of drug-using parents have these difficulties – see 'Resilience', p. 43.)

Partners and spouses of drug users are very vulnerable. They may be subjected to both physical and psychological abuse, constantly asked for money and emotionally blackmailed. Their levels of stress are likely to be very high, not least because being the partner of a drug abuser brings its own problems – the drug user may, for example, own the home that his partner and children live in and it may be very difficult to get him out if the partner feels she is unable to cope. A study of 153 male drug addicts in Spain found that six out of ten had directed some form of violence towards their partners, including personal control, sexual abuse and social isolation. A study of partners of alcoholics found that they were more likely to experience victimization, injury, mood disorders and anxiety disorders, and to have other health problems, and pointed out that these problems 'go beyond [alcoholism's] well-documented association with domestic violence'.

So having an addict in the family can have a huge impact on both the immediate carers – for example, parents who feel that it is their responsibility to help the addict – and other members of the family, who may not be directly involved in the drive to get the addict 'clean' but are nevertheless very aware of what is going on.

It takes completely centre-stage in our family. It dominates everything from whether we all get together for family lunch to whether we can go on holiday. Even in daily conversation with my parents there's never a family interaction that isn't in some way dominated by his problems. My mum comes to visit my children and she finds it really hard to turn her phone off or to completely disconnect because of the possibility that something will be going on for him. She finds it really hard to just switch off from his problems, I think.   (Lisa)

It has a dire, dire effect on the family. My wife doted on him. She's become quite reclusive now. She still hasn't come to terms with it, I don't think. It's a motherly thing, isn't it? The mother–son bond. My other son is two years older and absolutely no trouble whatsoever. Wouldn't take a paracetamol for a headache. But he's had to endure all this as much as us, even though he doesn't live with us. He's had to experience some of it. He told me that he felt like a bit of an outsider because all the attention was all going towards the other one. I understand that, obviously. Our argument would be that you didn't need the support, you weren't causing any trouble. We're grateful for that but we have to give our attention where it's needed – albeit we discovered we were being foolish to do it. (Alan)

Abusive behaviour

Not all drug users are abusive. It's believed that drug abuse doesn't necessarily cause domestic abuse – but it can make it worse. If you are living with a drug user who is not violent, you may not see yourself as being subject to 'abuse'. But abuse can take many forms, psychological as well as physical. The following examples could all be indications that your family member is abusing you:

- Isolation: stopping you seeing friends and family; confiscating your phone; preventing you from going to work; or telling members of your social circle that you don't want to see them any more.
- Humiliation: insulting, belittling or mocking you in front of others, including your children; telling you that you are worthless.
- Jealousy: checking your phone, computer or email; following you; insisting that you are flirting with other people or having affairs.
- Fear: making you or your children afraid in any way; threatening you or your children.
- Blame: insisting that he only behaves this way because the drugs or alcohol are forcing him to do it.
- Threats: threatening that your children will be taken away; that you will be seen as a bad parent; that you will be arrested.
- Force: using physical violence on you or your children; forcing you to have sex against your will or perform sex acts that you don't want to do; making you do things that you don't want to do.
- Financial abuse: stealing money; denying you access to money; demanding money, savings or benefits such as Child Benefit or a pension.

It can be very hard to admit that you are a victim of domestic abuse. It still, sadly, carries a stigma. But, like drug abuse, domestic abuse does not discriminate and happens in households across the social spectrum. Any abuse within the family can have a dire effect on those involved, even on those who are not the abuser's direct target – for example, children who are aware of and witness the abuse of a parent. If you think that you are a victim of domestic abuse, you should seek help as soon as possible. (See 'Useful addresses' for more details on help and advice.)

Your health

Stress is not just some imaginary condition suffered by overworked office managers who are feeling a bit underappreciated. Nor is it a 'fake' condition invoked by people trying to get a few weeks off work to redecorate the lounge – whatever the press would have you believe. Stress can have very real physical and mental effects, including insomnia and depression. The stress of coping with a drug addict in the family is enormous. Add it to the everyday burdens of holding down a job, looking after children or caring for older members of your family and it's hardly surprising that your own health, both physical and mental, will suffer.

But because of all these demands on your time, you may find that you are neglecting your own health, pushing potential problems to the back of your mind because they don't seem as important as those of the drug user and all the other people you have to look after. You may feel that you simply don't have the time to go to the doctor. You may feel that you have to be strong for your family, that you shouldn't complain. You may not want to be a worry to those in your family who are looking to you for support. But however you decide to tackle this problem, you will find it easier if you are physically and mentally healthy. It is worth taking time out to consider how you feel and to seek help if you need it – and perhaps even if you feel you don't.

Some common health problems experienced by families of drug addicts

- *Having problems with sleep.* You may find that you are too worried to sleep if the user is out and hasn't returned. You may lie awake waiting for a call, or be up all night dealing with a situation caused by the user. You might have nightmares when you do sleep, or you might even find that you are sleeping too much and finding it difficult to get out of bed in the morning.
- *Experiencing overwhelming negative feelings.* These may be feelings such as not being able to concentrate at home when you're doing things that used to relax you, or not being able to concentrate at work. You might feel panicky or have panic attacks, and you may even have suicidal thoughts or depression (see p. 21).
- *Relying on substances yourself.* Relying on substances to help you through this difficult time doesn't mean that you're taking illegal drugs, but you might start smoking again, for example, or smoke more than you did. You might start drinking to stop the stress, or eat too much or too little. All these activities can in turn affect your health.
- *Experiencing physical symptoms.* You may experience actual physical symptoms such as feeling sick, having headaches, diarrhoea or a change in your usual bowel movement patterns, general aches and pains or asthma.

If you are having any of these problems, don't push them to the back of your mind or tell yourself that they don't matter – seek help before they overwhelm you. However you choose to deal with the user in your family, you'll be in a better position to make decisions if you are well.

Tips for dealing with stress
- Take time for yourself. Try and find some space and time where you're not thinking about the family situation. Don't give up on hobbies or seeing friends. Something as simple as leaving the house for a walk or going swimming can give you some room to

breathe. It's not a betrayal of your loved one not to spend every waking moment thinking about him – it's actually a positive thing which will help make you stronger for your family.

- Eat healthily and regularly. Again, this will make you healthier, stronger and better able to cope.
- Try not to use food, alcohol or cigarettes as a coping mechanism. They may seem to work in the short term but in the long term you could be storing up health problems for yourself.
- Investigate relaxation techniques such as deep breathing and meditation to help you calm down in high-pressure situations. This may seem ridiculous – how is breathing going to help you solve your problem? – but again, it's all about making it easier for you to cope with the problem.
- Get regular exercise. Exercise has been shown to reduce stress levels and will give you a well-earned break. Choose something you enjoy – it could be as simple as a walk, a bike ride, a salsa class or a swim – and you'll be more motivated to keep it up regularly.
- Spend time with positive people who love and support you. If you feel that your friends and family are not supportive, find a support group or even an internet forum where people will understand your situation. There is always someone out there who has been through what you are going through.

Depression

Depression is a serious illness and a very real risk for those dealing with the stress of having a drug abuser within the family. It is known that depression can be triggered by events. It can be hard to work out the difference between 'everyday' sadness and depression, so it is worth knowing the symptoms. It's a complex disorder and these can vary considerably from person to person, so the following is just a guide:

- disturbed sleep patterns or problems getting to sleep
- feelings of hopelessness and helplessness
- taking no pleasure in things that you used to enjoy, like hobbies
- crying a lot

- feeling guilty
- thinking about harming yourself, or suicide
- a reduced sex drive
- lack of motivation.

If you think you might have depression, it's important to get professional help as soon as possible. Don't be afraid to speak to your GP about treatment, which could be counselling or anti-depressants. You may feel worried about the possibility of being prescribed anti-depressants and want to avoid taking any kind of drug. That's a completely valid concern. However, anti-depressants can be a great help to some people and there is no shame whatsoever in using a drug for its intended purpose. Your GP will be able to advise you on the right medication for you, and will be able to answer any questions or concerns that you have about possible addiction. A GP is also a great first point of contact for support services in your area (see 'Finding support for yourself and your family', p. 25).

> I got into a better place to deal with things, deal with Steve, and I became a volunteer worker. I was a family support worker. But after two and a half years it was difficult at times doing that, because I was working with addicts and they were telling me how they felt when they needed – they said it's not just the drugs, it's the whole thing of going out, stealing the money, buying the heroin, preparing it, you know – so I became very aware of what Steve was doing. And that was hard. After two and a half years I had a breakdown. My husband had an accident, my mother had an accident, I had both of them at home on crutches. It was depression. I just couldn't cope with anything. I sat with a hot water bottle all day. I went to bed, didn't want to get up. It was just a total meltdown. Luckily, I had a good GP who referred me to a psychologist, where I got help.
>
> (Miriam)

For more information on where to get help with depression, see 'Useful addresses'.

Dealing with your feelings

We've talked briefly in this chapter about the kind of negative feelings you may experience – guilt, fear, shame, helplessness, stress and worry. Here, we'll discuss positive ways of dealing with these feelings which you can use yourself and talk about with other family members.

Asserting yourself

Having a drug addict in the family can give you a profound feeling of loss of control. You cannot control what your family member does. You may feel utterly helpless to deal with him. There is, unfortunately, no way of controlling what an adult does. So concentrate on what you can control – your own actions. One way of doing this is through assertiveness, and a big part of assertiveness is learning how to say no.

Like all behavioural techniques, assertiveness comes with practice. Initially, you may find it extremely hard to say no. Don't suddenly try to put all these suggestions into practice straight away. Think about the kind of situations that might arise in which you might need these techniques, and try them out when you feel ready.

- Don't be afraid to say what you feel. Your own thoughts, feelings and opinions are important. Don't deny them. Use 'I' rather than 'you' to avoid apportioning blame – for example, rather than 'You come in at five o'clock in the morning and wake the whole house up', you might say: 'I feel very worried when I don't know what time you're going to be home', or 'I really hate it when I don't know where you are and I have to wait up for you.'
- Express your own needs and desires. They don't automatically come second to everyone else's.
- Practise saying no without feeling guilty. Saying yes when you don't really mean it or you don't really want to do something adds to that feeling of loss of control – you are being forced into doing something you don't want to. Saying no will help you take back that control over your own life. Again, you can't

control what the addict does, but you can control what you do or don't do.

- Say what you want and what you don't want. Set your own goals and work out what your own priorities are. Make these clear to the person you are talking to. Again, this is all about seeking more control over your own life and that of your family.

- Assertiveness can be seen as aggression. It's a powerful tool, so use it wisely. You may feel that it's better not to assert yourself in some situations, and this is fine. Only you can decide where assertiveness will be appropriate and where it might make a situation worse. In many cases, being aggressive towards the user won't help and may even make him more determined to continue with his behaviour.

- How you present yourself physically can help assertiveness to be more effective. Making eye contact with the person you are talking to and keeping your voice calm and collected can help get your message across.

When you're using assertiveness, the following techniques will help you:

1 *Behavioural rehearsal.* Practise what you want to say. (Don't feel silly doing it in front of a mirror – this will also help you with your physical presentation.)

2 *Repeated assertion* – the 'broken record' technique. Saying something again and again will help your message get through and keep the discussion to the point.

3 *Fogging.* Acknowledge the view of the other person, agreeing that it may contain some truth, but stick to your chosen course of action.

4 *Negative enquiry.* This allows expression of feelings to improve communication, for example: 'So you really believe that I don't care?'

5 *Negative assertion.* This allows comfort with your own negatives and reduces your critic's hostility. For example: 'Yes, you are right. I don't seem to care sometimes.'

6 *Workable compromise.* Agree to this only when you feel that your

position overall will not be compromised and no precedent is being set.

Dealing with anger

Anger is normal. It's a normal, understandable response to a threat – the well-known 'fight or flight' response. When we're angry, our blood pressure rises and our heart rate increases. We become more tense – you may feel that tension in a particular place in your body, such as your jaw or your shoulders. Repressing your anger can make you feel even more stressed, so it's worth exploring some positive ways of dealing with it.

- Change your environment. Go for a walk, or leave the room. Give yourself a break from whatever is making you angry.
- Work out exactly why you are angry. Are you angry because you are scared? Or because a rule has been broken and you feel as if you have lost control? Is your anger a symptom of something deeper?
- Remember your 'I' statements. Say what is making you angry and why.
- Think about how you deal with stress and look at the tips on pp. 20–1.
- Remember that being assertive and being aggressive are two very different things. Stay assertive, not aggressive. Aggression may just make the situation worse.
- Remember your positives. It can be useful to have a 'mantra' to repeat to yourself when you become angry: for example, 'I am able to make good choices, based on what's best for everyone in the long term.'

Finding support for yourself and your family

The following information is intended as a guide only to help you decide what kind of approach – if any – you would like to follow. There is no 'right way' as every family and every situation is different. It cannot be stressed enough that if you decide to investigate any kind of therapy, you should ensure that you contact a fully qualified family therapist. For more information on how to find a family therapist, see 'Useful addresses' at the end of the book.

> We did a survey with our clients and they said that it takes an average of five years to contact us. It's a long time but that seems to be about the average. I think that most families try and deal with the situation themselves. From personal experience, I know that you just try absolutely everything and it's only when you come to the end of your tether that you start to think: 'We've tried this, we've tried that, now what is there left to try? Maybe we need to ask for some help, advice or guidance with this.' We do also get people coming whose son or daughter has tried drugs for the first time and they are thinking: my God, how do I play this? They don't want to alienate their son or daughter but they don't want them to be doing drugs. So we do get those initial ones. But generally, when people come to us it is a last resort.
>
> (Jane, support network director)

Support and 'fellowship' groups

Support groups can be very helpful. Usually these consist of people like you, who meet to exchange information, to discuss any questions relating to their situation and to support each other emotionally. Support groups can be accessed via your local substance abuse services.

There are also 'fellowship groups' for families, such as Families Anonymous (FA). FA follows the 12-step approach pioneered by Alcoholics Anonymous and its groups for the families of alcoholics, Al-Anon and Alateen. These groups use an approach which centres on the powerlessness of family members. You did not cause your family member's problem, you cannot control it, and the suggestion is generally to use 'loving detachment' – not commenting on the drug use or its consequences, making it clear that you will offer no help, and not attempting to influence the drug user in any way, whether that's pleading with him to go for treatment or giving him money for a fix. This approach, again, is suitable for some family members and not for others.

There is not a great deal of research into how effective support groups are for families of drug users, but research into Al-Anon has shown that wives of problem drinkers who attended the group suffered less from depression, family conflict and anger.

However, it's also recognized that there are certain barriers for family members seeking help via any kind of support group.

Stigma

Admitting that a family member is a drug addict still carries an enormous stigma and shame. It can take years for you to come to terms with the drug addiction, let alone be in a position where you feel able to talk about it with other people. You may simply not like the idea of ever sharing your experiences and feel that this approach would not work for you. You might also be worried about being seen leaving or attending the place where the meeting's being held.

Availability

Provision of support groups across the UK varies widely from area to area and there may simply not be anything available where you are. If this is the case, 'Useful addresses' lists several telephone helplines where you can get advice and support.

Practicalities

You may have young children and be unable to leave them to attend a support group in the evening. Those living in rural areas without transport may have difficulties in attending evening groups as buses or trains may not be running then.

Fear

Many of us have a very clichéd view of support groups. They are usually portrayed on TV and in films as intimidating, highly emotional, confessional sessions, in which the affected person invariably stands up and pours out his life story to claps and cheers before swearing to devote his life to God. Needless to say, this is not an accurate picture of support groups! However, it's perfectly valid to have these concerns. Few of us enjoy the prospect of 'opening up' in front of strangers. If you do decide to access a support group and have concerns about this, it may be worth calling ahead and asking exactly what's involved.

> My parents went to something like Narcotics Anonymous – maybe it was that. I remember being a teenager and going with them to some sort of support group for families of people with drug problems. And it was the first time I'd ever talked about it. I kind of wasn't expecting to have to say anything. But I remember someone saying in the group did I want to say anything and I remember it being a really traumatic experience – I was the first to speak and I fell apart and I found it very unhelpful. That was quite a seminal point for me to detach from some of those structures that are supposed to help.
>
> (Lisa)

> Don't be frightened to ask for help. I found my family support group to be invaluable. The help I got off them was just amazing. There's a lot more drug support now for families. Your GP will signpost you to local ones.
>
> (Miriam)

> We have had no support as a family. There is none that we are aware of. I've had plenty of discussions with drugs counsellors. But they are always those who have called here for an appointment with David and he hasn't turned up. So I've always been left with the drugs counsellor, chatting to them. But frankly, some of them were just as bad as he was. I know some of them were ex-addicts and I think some of them were still using, even though they were drugs counsellors.
>
> (Alan)

> People do think they are alone a lot of the time. Four of us from the same area found each other via an internet forum. We started my own group because if you're involved with other people, you can always talk together. It just makes you feel better to sit down and sometimes we laugh about some of the horrendous things that have happened to us all. Other people might find it a bit sick, some of the things we laugh about, but that's how we deal with it.
>
> (Carly)

We had no support apart from one very helpful GP. I never felt the need to get support and my parents would never have joined a support group or anything like that. They are just not that sort of person. They are from a generation that doesn't talk about its problems and that's fine, support groups don't work for everyone. But the GP was brilliant – she never judged my brother.   (Marcus)

What really happens inside a support group – a family support worker's insight

The film version is very different from the reality. Support groups are facilitated. They are not self-help. We have two trained volunteers in each group. Some are also trained counsellors who offer their services free of charge because they want to help, but also it's good for their personal development. But volunteers are from all walks of life.

It's a safe place where you can talk about things. We don't repeat stuff outside the room. We always have decent tea and coffee and we always have music playing when people walk in the room so there's not a deathly silence. Some venues are better than others – some are like lounges and others aren't! We try to make it friendly and informal.

We have a 'care and share' where the facilitator goes round to each person and if they want to share, they can. If they don't, they don't have to. They might want to share what happened the last time they came. There's an opportunity for the group to feed back to them about what they've heard with advice, support and ideas on how to move forward.

Other groups are run in different ways but ours is very group-led. The group decides what happens in the room. For example, the same issue might keep coming up – housing, for example. Support for someone who wants to keep the family in the same home, or how to get someone to leave the home. So the facilitator might say: 'Quite a lot of you have brought up housing issues. So would it be helpful to get a guest speaker along to talk about that particular issue, or for you to pick their brains?' If the group says that would be helpful, then great; if not, it's their decision. The group takes the lead and they might have someone come and talk to them about that. Or maybe someone to talk about what drug or alcohol treatment entails.

What we do is always offer people a number of options. So ideas, really, of what other people have done in similar circumstances. Then we encourage the client to talk through those options, positive and negative. Talk through the kind of things that might happen if they follow through with options. We don't use terms like 'rock bottom' or 'tough love'. People are individuals. Nobody is going to get told, 'You have to throw them out.' We don't run that way at all. We always say, 'Well, what are the options? If you did ask him or her to leave, what would happen? How would you feel? What would be the consequences of that? If he was to stay, what would the options and consequences be?' Ultimately it's the client's decision. We would talk through the options that other families might have put in place in similar circumstances. We would never tell people what to do.

Family support drop-in centres

Drop-in centres are usually designed to be an easy first point of contact with support services. You probably won't need an appointment, though you will usually be able to phone ahead and get one if you'd like one. Some are open outside normal office hours as well as during the day, so if you are working they are still accessible for you to go to after work.

Drop-in centre services vary around the country, but they will usually provide:

- some form of counselling, individually or with a group;
- practical help and advice on, for example, needle disposal, legal problems and questions, health problems;
- information and advice on all aspects of drug taking;
- information on different kinds of treatment options;
- a cup of tea and a friendly non-judgemental ear.

What you might expect from a drop-in centre – a family support worker's insight

A drop-in centre is quite informal. When people first arrive, obviously we make them as welcome as possible. The first thing we do is provide refreshments. A cup of tea is always a good icebreaker. Decent refreshments are vital! The other thing we do is ask them to sign their name in the visitors' book, but we only ask for their first name and they can give any name they like – we don't ask for an address, they can ignore that. It's just about fire regulations – we just need a name in the book.

Then we go through exactly what we do. We talk through that this is a safe place where they can talk in confidence about a friend or relative's drink or drug abuse. We don't judge, we do our best to support. We hold any information they give us in confidence unless we hear that someone is at risk of serious harm, in which case we may have to take it further, but we will always keep the person fully informed. That's our safeguarding policy.

We always say that this is a free service. You can use it as many times as you need, we're here on Tuesday night or whenever it is, and refreshments are provided. People know exactly what they're coming to. They know what to expect. They know they won't have to pay for a support session, or for the refreshments, because sometimes little things like that make people feel quite ill at ease, not knowing if they have to pay for something or not knowing how much tea costs. It's quite important.

Here's an example of a typical contact. We had a call to our helpline yesterday – a 20-year-old girl worried about her mum's drinking. She gave us permission to get an advisor to call her back. He called her and said, 'Hi, my name's Tom, I'm going to be at the drop-in tonight. I understand you're thinking about coming down. Shall I meet you outside so we can walk in together and I can introduce myself?' It broke the ice a bit and now she's got a name, someone who described himself to her, so she could look out for him. They went in together. He made her a cup of tea, went through all the processes, and they sat down together and he had his colleague on call in case he needed her. She's a young girl, around the same age, so she could pop in and say, 'Are you all right, have you got everything you need?' So if she didn't click with him there was someone else she could talk to. We've got a range of 30 volunteers, so we do try and match people of similar age and background.

They spent an hour together talking through all her concerns about her mum, what she does to support herself – who looks after her, where does she go, what does she do to protect herself? He made sure that she didn't leave without the telephone helpline, and that she understood that it's open every day until ten at night. If she gets the answerphone she can leave a message, they'll call her back and be discreet about it – all these things are really important. It might be that she gets signposts to another service, like a counselling service or something else.

Once the person has built up trust, then she might say that she could do with listening to how other people are coping in similar situations. So Tom would support her into a support group, if that's what she felt she wanted. But he'd always be reviewing her support options.

A lot of people come not really knowing what to expect but they do expect to be given help and information on drugs and alcohol and to be able to explore the options of what they could do. Some people say, 'I thought you were going to tell me I should do this and that', but they get that from everyone else – their brother, their sister, their GP. And we don't feel it's our place to say that. Our place is maybe to challenge some of their perceptions but in a way that is not judgemental.

3

Ways of coping

Every family is different. There is no right or wrong answer when you are seeking to know how you can deal with the situation of having a problematic drug user in the family. In this chapter, we'll discuss the various options open to you. It's then up to you to decide how you want to move forward.

The internet has proved a fantastic resource for information sharing, particularly for families who feel very isolated. However, it's important to remember that however miraculous a family's tale of recovery sounds, it is not your family. Only you can make the decision that is right for yourself and your family. Do not allow yourself to feel pressured into doing something simply because it has worked for someone else, and don't allow your own coping techniques to be belittled simply because they are different from someone else's.

Accepting the situation

You've probably heard the 'serenity prayer' – 'God, grant me the serenity to accept the things I cannot change, courage to change the things I can, and wisdom to know the difference.' It's used by many organizations, such as Alcoholics Anonymous. Although it may seem trite, there's a real core of truth there and it's a good starting point to think about how you will move forward.

You may feel that one of the things you can change is the behaviour of the addict in your family, and certainly family support has been found to be a factor in the success of treatment. However, when it comes down to it, there is only so much you can do. How you can best help your family member into treatment, during treatment and beyond is discussed in Chapter 5. This chapter will focus on helping you identify the things that you can't change.

Acceptance is a long-term way of thinking. It doesn't happen instantly and most of us go through a recognized process:

- Denial – 'This isn't happening to me'.
- Anger – finding someone to blame, offering ultimatums, using threats.
- Bargaining – 'If you must do this, then do it my way'.
- Depression – a normal and important part of the process which allows deeper understanding.
- Acceptance – emotional detachment (with love) and objectivity. The user is allowed his consequences. The family member begins to live in a new reality and takes care of him or herself.

It's likely that you will recognize your own behaviour in some of these stages.

> My parents have gone through probably 20 years of different things – support groups or going to different places for help. They've tried everything. They've offered to pay for him to go to places like that – the Priory – they would do anything, I think. I don't think there's anything they haven't tried. But until he chooses to make changes in his life there's really nothing they can do. They're in this cycle of constantly feeling helpless, trying to do something, going back to the point they were at – until he makes that choice, they can't really do anything.
>
> (Lisa)

Identify your coping strategies

Exactly what is 'coping'? The dictionary defines it as 'to struggle or deal with, especially on fairly even terms or with some degree of success' and 'to face and deal with responsibilities, problems, or difficulties, especially successfully or in a calm or adequate manner'. Perhaps you might feel some of the synonyms to be more apt – 'to wrestle', 'to strive', 'to persevere'. How well you are 'coping' is all relative. You may feel that you are coping well if you have just managed to get through a day without crying. Or you may feel that truly coping involves a higher degree of detachment. Whatever your perception, you will have found your own way of 'coping'.

We all have different ways of coping with stress, and over time you may find certain things work for you and certain things don't. You may not even be aware that you have these strategies, and you may not call them 'coping strategies'. They could be anything from actual activities (going for a walk) to things that you find yourself thinking in times of stress ('I cannot control my family member's behaviour and what is happening now is not my fault'). If you know what helps you cope, you can then summon up these resources when you need them the most.

When you're identifying these strategies, consider:

- Even when your loved one is using drugs, what is it that stops you from feeling completely overwhelmed by your feelings?
- How do you switch off from all these pressures?
- What is it like when you say to yourself that you cannot think or worry any more?
- What do you say to yourself when you can't be bothered to worry any more?

The 'stress-strain-coping' model

The stress-strain-coping model is laid out by Jim Orford, Alex Copello, Richard Velleman and Lorna Templeton in their 2010 study, published in the journal *Drugs: Education, Prevention and Policy*, 'Family members affected by a close relative's addiction: The stress-strain-coping-support model'.

It sounds rather mathematical and impersonal, but what it seeks to do is extremely useful. It tries to provide a way of understanding what the families of drug users go through. The theory runs as follows: living with a drug addict in the family is hugely stressful. This stress then leads to strain, which can produce psychological and physical symptoms, discussed in more detail in Chapter 2.

The amount of strain that the carer is under depends on two factors: coping and social support. How a carer chooses to cope can make him or her feel worse or better. Likewise, the quality of support provided by friends, other family members and health professionals can either increase or decrease the amount of strain the carer is under. In order to reduce the strain, the carer can either try to reduce the amount of stress he or she is under, or can seek out new and more helpful ways of coping or a more helpful support network.

How does this help you? It suggests that thinking about how you cope will help you work out how you can reduce your levels of strain.

As the study says:

> Stress-coping models . . . conceive of certain sets of conditions that people face in their everyday lives as constituting seriously stressful circumstances or conditions of adversity which are often longstanding . . . A central idea is that people facing such conditions have the capacity to 'cope' with them much as one would attempt to cope with any difficult or complex 'task' in life. That incorporates the idea of being active in the face of adversity, of effective problem solving, of being an agent in one's own destiny, of *not* being powerless.

Do you have a 'coping position'?

What follows is a useful description of three 'coping positions' identified in a 1998 study of the structures of families coping with substance abuse by Orford and colleagues, 'Tolerate, engage or withdraw: A study of the structure of families coping with alcohol and drug problems in South West England and Mexico City'.

Each one has its advantages and disadvantages. Looking at these strategies which carers commonly use – in many cases without actually making a conscious decision to act that way – may help you to identify the way you are dealing with your situation and help you think about whether or not it is working for you.

The *engaged* coper feels responsible for the user. She feels that she should be able to change his behaviour. She feels angry, hurt and responsible for the user. She may impose 'rules', keep a watchful eye on his behaviour, check his room for drugs or his mobile phone for dealers' numbers. She may try to get him a job or organize his life in some other way. Although she feels that at least she is doing something positive, she also feels very stressed, exhausted and resentful that she is having to keep tabs on her family member in this way.

The *tolerant* coper may feel guilty and powerless to deal with the situation. He may feel that others don't understand his child. He may give the user money to spend on drugs, or cover up for his failure to turn up at work or for a counselling appointment. This way of coping means that the coper avoids conflict but may feel that the user is taking advantage of him.

The *withdrawn* coper will try to put distance between herself and the user and leave the user to look after himself. She may feel either hurt or self-reliant. She may avoid seeing the user as much as possible and feel that it's better if they are apart. This way of coping can stop carers becoming too involved, but they may also feel bad for rejecting the user.

> I didn't ring him, didn't speak to him, didn't offer him any help. I just didn't want to know him. He'd be round my place, asking for money and I told him no, I never gave him a thing. I felt very cold when I did that, and very guilty, but I didn't want him dragging me down. In a way, I felt quite proud of myself for not being 'emotional' like my parents were. I was the strong one, they were the weak ones. (Marcus)

Am I co-dependent?

You might have heard that families of drug addicts are 'co-dependent'. Like a lot of words which started in psychology and are now commonly used by lay people, it can be misused and misunderstood. ('Schizophrenic' is a good example of this – it's now used to mean a contradictory attitude towards something, as if the person has a 'split personality', when in fact schizophrenia is nothing of the sort.) So it's worth taking a little time to understand what we mean when we say 'co-dependent', as it means a lot of different things to different people.

'Co-dependency' isn't listed in DSM, which as we've seen is the main diagnostic manual used by psychologists and psychiatrists. So you can't get an official diagnosis of co-dependency. It is, however, a recognized concept within psychology and addiction therapy and one that has been studied, and is a term you are likely to hear if you attend Al-Anon or Families Anonymous.

The Merriam-Webster dictionary defines co-dependency as 'a psychological condition or a relationship in which a person is controlled or manipulated by another who is affected with a pathological condition (such as an addiction to alcohol or heroin)'. The broader definition is 'dependence on the needs of or control by others'. Basically, the co-dependent person is a 'caretaker' who fulfils the needs of others before his or her own to an excessive, unhealthy degree. It is possible to have co-dependent relationships within the family, in a circle of friends or at work.

In terms of drug addiction within the family, the theory runs that the co-dependent person then becomes the 'enabler' for the addict. He or she will 'indulge' the addict's behaviour by, for example, buying his drugs or giving him money, and putting up with unreasonable behaviour. The co-dependant may also suffer from patterns of:

- denial – for example, having difficulty identifying how you are feeling, labelling others with your negative traits, a lack of empathy;
- low self-esteem – for example, having difficulty making decisions, being unable to ask others to meet your needs or desires;
- compliance – for example, excessive loyalty, remaining in harmful situations for too long, compromising your own values to avoid rejection or anger;
- control – for example, believing that most people are incapable of taking care of themselves, pretending to agree with others to get what you want;
- avoidance – for example, believing that displays of emotion are a sign of weakness, suppressing your needs to avoid feeling vulnerable.

These are just a few examples of patterns that co-dependants may fall into. A full list of the patterns of co-dependency can be found on the Co-Dependents Anonymous website – see 'Useful addresses' for more details.

There is some disagreement among experts surrounding co-dependency and how helpful a concept it can be to a person dealing with addiction within the family. Identifying as co-dependent has certainly helped many people deal with their situation and has given them a framework, a strategy for coping and moving on. But others find the label stigmatizing and feel that their own 'co-dependency' means that they are to blame for the actions of their partners. The co-dependant, it is implied, is the person at fault, and recovering and recognizing co-dependency means admitting to your own inadequacies – even possibly to the extent that you have 'sought out' a drug user to 'look after'.

If you feel that investigating co-dependency further would help you, I have included information on further reading at the end of the book.

He lives in the same town as my parents. Probably about half an hour away. But he's very – again, this is maybe more related to his mental health issues than the drugs – dependent on them. They probably have quite a co-dependent relationship in that because there's nothing they can really do to help him, they end up doing his washing or doing his food shopping and stuff like that. I think they are probably trapped into quite a co-dependent relationship.   (Lisa)

Identifying the support around you

It may be that not everyone in your family agrees with your particular stance on the user in your family. Try to keep communication going. It can help to sit down together, without the user present, and try to work out exactly how you feel and what you are going to do as a unit. Presenting a united front can help a great deal. A lack of communication may lead to other family members feeling left out.

The thing that's been hard but really important for us to do is to hold it together as a family. There's been times where I think things were really chaotic and out of control and he didn't have a diagnosis and we didn't know what was wrong with him, and he was doing all sorts of drugs and in trouble with the police the whole time. We didn't sit down and go: this is happening to our family, what shall we do, how shall we support each other? We all dealt with it in our own ways. There have been points where we were forced to deal with it as a family. I remember sitting down with my parents when we went away on holiday one year and he went nuts – and the three of us crying our eyes out and talking through the stuff – what can we do? How can we cope? At that point it didn't feel helpful – I found it really awkward – but there's been quite consistent stages ever since then, maybe once a year, we'll talk really openly and candidly. And that being there for one another as a family and trying to contain the way that we feel together has been really helpful.

(Lisa)

You may find the attitudes of your wider social network differing dramatically. Some will want to help. Others may not appreciate how you feel and won't understand why you are taking particular decisions ('Why don't you just throw him out?' or 'Why did you throw him out?'). Try to work out who will be supportive, who will be helpful and who won't. The stigma of drug use means that it can be very hard to admit these problems to friends and family. But having that wider social support can make all the difference. If you think it would be useful to talk more about your problems to people who can provide support, do so.

When you can no longer cope

It may be that you feel you have done everything possible to help your family member and that the time has come to ask him to leave the family home. You may also have decided to stop all contact. You may feel that it is now time for you to separate your life and your family's lives from that of the user. Perhaps he has become aggressive or is stealing from you. Perhaps the stress and worry of living with a drug addict have become too much for you. Perhaps you are concerned about the toll that the addiction has taken on other family members.

This is never an easy decision. It may have been something that others have been pressing you to do and you have tried to put off. Or it may be something that you have been wanting to do for a long time. However you feel about making the final break, it's important that you think about it carefully before you take that step. It is a decision that only you and your family can make. Try not to feel pressured one way or the other. It's easy for well-meaning friends to tell you what they think you should do – but they are not the ones who will have to actually do it. They are not the ones who will have to live with the drug user if you decide that he should stay, and they are not the ones who will have to make the decision to ask their child to leave the family home, or tell their child that they will no longer talk to him on the phone or allow him to visit.

Some things you may want to consider before ending the relationship:

- Have I done everything I can to help the user?
- Have my efforts made any impact on him?
- What will be the consequences if I do end the relationship – both good and bad?
- What kind of future can I see for myself and my family if I do end the relationship?
- What is the best way to go about ending the relationship?
- What kind of practical things do I need to consider when ending the relationship? (For example, does he have any legal right to stay in my home? Is he likely to become violent? Might I need support from the police or from a social worker?)

The only sound piece of advice we received, which we didn't act upon for some time, was to get him out of our lives. That is a very hard thing to say. He is my son, at the end of the day. But I don't think anyone in my situation can be hard enough. You have to be absolutely firm and resolute. You have to forget that they are your son or daughter. You have to be completely ruthless with them. Wipe them out of your lives. Unless they show signs of actually wanting and responding to support, you must wash your hands of them. Otherwise you will have a life of misery. It was a very hard decision to take. I still wonder now – we haven't spoken to him for a year but we still wonder whether this was the wisest thing to do. But when you look at the practical reasons why we came to that decision, then yes. Common sense would tell you that. You can't do it. Bear in mind that we are looking after his son full time. He is a constant reminder. Thankfully we are here to provide for him. But you would think that there would be some level of gratitude and respect as recompense for that, but no. I would say just be as ruthless as you possibly can. And a bit more.   (Alan)

My husband, I don't know whether it's a male thing, but he was more, right, I'm finished with him, that's the end of it. I wasn't. I had a bit more empathy with him. I think it was being a mother. He was my baby. To me, there was always hope. So it caused a lot of arguments between me and my husband. Invariably, my husband always said he'd been right, Steve would relapse again. There was no easy answer. There's not. Unless the user wants to help themselves, nothing is ever going to work. Steve was seeing a counsellor, having therapy, but it just continued in the same cycle and the same cycle of us helping, which, looking back, enabled him to continue. But he wasn't prepared to live by what we were asking. Our rules. It was our house. Some nights he would come and knock at the door, be with one of his friends, totally off his head. One time he came, he'd been beaten up and he was – his head – there was blood all over him. I cleaned him up and I had to send him back out into the night because I knew he was so heavily back into the drugs, he couldn't stay at home.   (Miriam)

I felt very strongly that my parents should throw him out and leave him to fend for himself. I told them that, several times. But they wouldn't. They said it was too big a risk and that they couldn't put a child of theirs on to the streets. At the time, I judged them very harshly. I actually think, now, that they made the right choice, to allow him to stay and help him – but it's easy to say that with hindsight. It could all have turned out very differently if he hadn't actually managed to kick the drugs.   (Marcus)

Resilience

The presence of a drug user within the family can bring so many associated problems – physical, mental and social – that it can be hard to see how your family will survive. But studies show that many family members aren't adversely affected by the user's behaviour, and there are factors within a family which can make a difference.

The question which sparked interest in resilience is: 'How can some people go through unimaginable trauma and emerge unscathed?' The concept is a much talked about subject in the field of 'positive psychology' and it's currently being used in everything from businesses to the British Army. As yet there has been little research done on resilience in the partners, parents and siblings of drug addicts, though much has been done on how children can develop resilience.

Velleman and Templeton's study 'Understanding and modifying the effects of parents' substance abuse on children', which I've already referred to (see p. 15), puts forward a list of possible protective factors that may help to develop resilience. It's worth mentioning that the authors do sound a note of caution:

> All strategies have potential associated risk; their success or levels of benefits are by no means guaranteed. This means that the processes that allow young people to become resilient may not all be totally positive, either in the short or the long term.
>
> (Velleman and Templeton 2007)

Velleman and Templeton point out, for example, that strategies which are effective when dealing with a younger child may be harmful in the long term. They cite a study which showed that detachment from family members whose 'domestic and emotional problems threaten to engulf them' is effective when used by a child who is otherwise powerless. However, as that child grows older, he or she may end up with relationship or attachment difficulties as a result.

Also, some factors can't be controlled or influenced – for example, other factors involved in the development of resilience include being raised in a small family and the individual personality of the child in question (see the following box for more factors) – but others may be within a concerned family member's personal remit, if that's a path you choose to take. In terms of children dealing with a parent's substance abuse, these 'protective' factors include the presence of a 'stable adult figure' and a 'close positive bond with at least one adult in a caring role', such as a grandparent or an older sibling. If you know that a child is suffering from a parent's drug abuse, this may be something that you can influence. You may be prepared to be that figure.

These 'protective' factors don't guarantee that the child will not be damaged by his or her experiences. But they do seem to lessen that risk. They encourage the development of resilient qualities, such as the child feeling in control of his or her life, higher self-esteem and the ability to deal with change.

Protective factors and resilience

Protective factors:

- The presence of a stable adult figure (usually not a substance misuser)
- Close positive bond with at least one adult in a caring role (e.g. parents, older siblings, grandparents)
- A good support network beyond this
- Little separation from the primary carer in the first year of life
- Parents' positive care style and characteristics
- Being raised in a small family
- Larger age gaps between siblings
- Engagement in a range of activities
- Individual temperament
- Positive opportunities at times of life transition
- Continuing family cohesion and harmony in the face of the misuse and its related effects (e.g. domestic violence, serious mental health problems).

Evidence of resilience that these protective factors encourage:

- Deliberate planning by the child that his or her adult life will be different
- High self-esteem and confidence
- Self-efficacy
- An ability to deal with change
- Skills and values that lead to good use of personal ability
- A good range of problem-solving skills
- Feeling that there are choices
- Feeling in control of his or her own life
- Previous experience of success and achievement.

(Velleman and Templeton 2007)

Thinking about resilience doesn't mean that you are somehow not 'allowed' to feel traumatized by your bad experiences, or that the people who aren't traumatized by unhappy childhoods or abusive marriages are somehow unfeeling or 'stronger' than others. It's more to do with trying to understand why some people are traumatized and some people aren't. If the last thing you are feeling right now is strong and resilient, don't feel bad or compare your experiences negatively to others ('She went through a much worse time than me and she's fine, therefore I'm weak and worthless'). Resilience doesn't just appear. It's a process, in many cases a very long process, which comes over time. Working with a counsellor in order to develop your resilience, work out your coping strategies and help you look forward might be something to consider.

As the American Psychological Association says in its booklet *The Road to Resilience*:

Being resilient does not mean that a person doesn't experience difficulty or distress. Emotional pain and sadness are common in people who have suffered major adversity or trauma in their lives. In fact, the road to resilience is likely to involve considerable emotional distress. Resilience is not a trait that people either have or do not have. It involves behaviors, thoughts, and actions that can be learned and developed in anyone.

It has affected me but I am also quite detached in some way. I'm more emotionally detached. I've never felt the need to seek counselling. When I was younger and still living at home it was much more difficult. I was so exposed to the pain that my parents experienced because of it. It was much harder then, and some of the times that they went to various support groups, some of that time I would have gone along with them to see if I was OK and needed any help. People do assume that you can't possibly be OK. But maybe it's part of the way I present that I'm a bit blithe about the whole thing. It seems to encourage people to push me and go 'Are you sure you're OK and not suppressing all that stuff?' But I never really felt the need for counselling. I think because I was so young. His problems really began when he was 12 or 13 so I was seven, so in some ways I didn't really have any other experience than having a brother with problems.   (Lisa)

I think we are both resilient. I like that word. We have both been through it and out the other side. I know that he has worked through his prob-lems and found better ways of dealing with them, and I know that he feels that whatever happens now, it can't possibly be as bad as his lowest points when he was addicted.   (Marcus)

4

Practical advice

As has been discussed in previous chapters, living with a drug user can be an introduction into a very different world. You may never before have considered the health implications of living with an injecting drug user, or wondered how to defuse a situation where someone is likely to become violent or aggressive. You may not have considered how to handle a situation where, for example, the drug user in your family has children of his or her own and you are concerned about their well-being. This chapter deals with the practical day-to-day considerations of living with a drug user. You may never need some of this knowledge, and you may never have to use some of it, but it's useful to have it in the background in case any of these issues arise.

Health concerns

The main health risks to non drug users in a household where there is a drug addict come from the dangers of blood-borne viruses. (However, if your family member is not injecting then this won't be a risk.) These viruses are transmitted from drug user to drug user when needles used by the infected person are shared. They can also be transmitted if a person injures himself with an infected needle, which is why it's important to take so much care when you're disposing of used needles.

There are three main blood-borne viruses you may be at risk from:

- Human immunodeficiency virus (HIV) is the virus which causes AIDS (Acquired Immune Deficiency Syndrome). There is no cure for AIDS but it can be treated. There is no vaccine.
- Hepatitis C (HCV) can be treated and cured. There is no vaccine available.

- Hepatitis B (HBV) can be treated, but a high proportion of sufferers (around nine out of ten) will become 'carriers' of the virus. As there is a vaccine available, it's a good idea to get yourself and family members vaccinated if you are living with an injecting drug user.

If you are worried about any of the above conditions, go to your GP or local clinic for testing. Testing is completely confidential. The earlier a condition is identified and treated, the more successful that treatment is likely to be.

What if my family member overdoses?

An accidental overdose can happen for a number of reasons:

- The user has not used a drug regularly in the period leading up to the overdose. This lowers his tolerance without him realizing it. Therefore, a smaller amount of the drug will have more of an effect on him than it did previously, leading to overdose.
- A 'batch' of the drug may be stronger than usual: it's impossible for the addict to determine exactly how strong a dose he is taking.
- The addict may have been drinking alcohol or taking other drugs which increase the risk of an adverse reaction.

Signs of an overdose

The following is a very basic guide, but bear in mind that symptoms will vary according to the drug taken. Of course, if you are concerned do not wait for other symptoms to appear but call an ambulance straight away.

- *Nervous system depressants and tranquillizers* such as barbiturates and benzodiazepines: lethargy and sleepiness, leading to unconsciousness; shallow breathing; weak, irregular or abnormally slow or fast pulse.
- *Stimulants and hallucinogens* including LSD, ecstasy, amphetamines (speed) and cocaine: excitable behaviour; wildness and frenzy; sweating; hallucinations; tremor of the hands.

- *Narcotics* including heroin and morphine: needle marks; slow, shallow breathing; unconsciousness; small pupils.
- *Solvents* including glue and lighter fluid: nausea and vomiting; hallucinations; headaches; possible unconsciousness; cardiac arrest (rare).

Treating an overdose until the ambulance arrives

Your aims are:

- to maintain breathing and circulation;
- to arrange removal to hospital.

If the casualty is conscious:

- Help him into a comfortable position.
- Ask him what he has taken.
- Reassure him while you talk to him.
- Dial 999 for an ambulance.
- Monitor and record vital signs – level of response, pulse and breathing – until medical help arrives.
- Look for evidence that might help to identify the drug, such as empty containers. Give these samples and containers to the paramedic or ambulance crew.

If the casualty becomes unconscious:

- Open the airway and check breathing.
- Be prepared to give chest compressions and rescue breaths if necessary.
- Place the casualty into the recovery position if he is unconscious but breathing normally.
- Dial 999 for an ambulance.
- *Do not* try to make the patient vomit.

The best way to learn how to resuscitate someone who is not breathing is to take a short first aid course. Please see 'Useful addresses' for more details.

A word on naloxone

Naloxone is an 'opioid antagonist' – it blocks the effect of opiate drugs such as heroin, codeine and methadone. It can be used to stop an opiate depressing the user's respiratory system and therefore it can be used to temporarily stop the effects of an overdose until an ambulance arrives. It doesn't work on drugs which aren't opiates, so it wouldn't work for cocaine, for example, or ketamine.

A recent study of 147 carer families in England, 89 per cent of whom were caring for a heroin addict, found that 49 per cent had experienced a family member having an overdose, and 21 per cent of the carers had witnessed an overdose. However, most families didn't know what to do in case of an overdose. Twenty-five per cent had received advice on overdose management and only 33 per cent were aware of naloxone. However, 88 per cent said that they would like training in overdose management, particularly in how to administer naloxone.

Naloxone is a controlled drug and you will need to be properly trained in order to access it. It's available to those caring for an addict and also to the user. Contact your local drug advisory service for more information.

How to minimize your health risk

In order to minimize the health risks to yourself and to other family members, never share any of the following with an injecting drug user:

- razors
- toothbrushes
- nail clippers
- scissors
- hair clippers
- cocaine straws (used to 'snort' cocaine')
- tattoo or piercing equipment.

You should also be aware of how to safely dispose of used injecting equipment ('sharps').

How to dispose of sharps

- You will need a sharps bin, a special bin which holds used needles safely. Never put used needles into the household waste. You can get a sharps bin on prescription from your GP, or from your local needle exchange. Make sure that you keep this bin in a safe place.
- Never directly handle a used syringe or needle. Don't try to re-sheath it. Always wear gloves and use a dustpan and brush or litter-picker tweezers to move the needle or syringe into the sharps bin. Put the needle straight into the bin – don't put it in another container first, such as a used drinks can or cardboard box.
- Never try to take a needle out of the sharps bin.
- Reduce the amount of time and risk it takes to move a sharp by taking the sharps bin to the needle, not the needle to the sharps bin.
- When the sharps bin is full, you can take it to your GP's surgery, a local pharmacy which provides a disposal service or the needle exchange, for safe disposal. Your local drug information service should be able to tell you what's available in your area.
- If you follow all the precautions listed above then your risk of a needle injury will be very low. However, if this does happen, immediately wash the wound with soap and water and go to A&E straight away. You will need to tell them exactly what happened.

Dealing with aggression

It is extremely frightening when a person becomes aggressive, and it goes without saying that you should call the police if you feel that the situation is getting out of control. Some drugs, such as cocaine and crack, can actually cause the user to become aggressive. However, any drug user can become aggressive in certain situations – for example, if he arrives home to find that his drugs have been

Am I at risk of arrest?

You may well be concerned about the possible legal consequence of having a drug user living in your home. It's a criminal offence to knowingly allow premises that you own, manage or have responsibility for to be used by any other person for:

- the administration or use of any controlled drug;
- the supply of any controlled drug;
- the production or cultivation of any controlled drug, such as growing cannabis.

This forms an amendment to Section 8 of the Misuse of Drugs Act, passed in 2001.

disposed of, or if he is attempting to force a family member to give him money for drugs.

You may find the following guidelines useful for dealing with aggression.

If the person becomes aggressive, assess the risks to yourself, the person and others. Ensure your own safety at all times so that you can continue to be an effective helper. If you feel unsafe, seek help from others. Do not stay with the person if your safety is at risk. Remain as calm as possible and try to de-escalate the situation with the following techniques:

- Talk in a calm, non-confrontational manner.
- Speak slowly and confidently with a gentle, caring tone of voice.
- Try not to provoke the person; refrain from speaking in a hostile or threatening manner and avoid arguing with him.
- Use positive words (such as 'stay calm') instead of negative words (such as 'don't fight') which may cause the person to overreact.
- Consider taking a break from the conversation to allow the person a chance to calm down.
- Try to provide the person with a quiet environment away from noise and other distractions.
- If inside, try to keep the exits clear so that the person does not

feel penned in, and so that you and others can get away easily if needed.
- If violence has occurred, seek appropriate emergency assistance.

When children are involved

Living with a drug abuser can have very serious consequences for children. Not only are they susceptible to the health risks described above, but they may suffer if the parent is incapable of looking after the child and meeting his or her needs. It is known that children of drug abusers who are unable to parent properly are more likely to become drug addicts themselves. They are also more likely to suffer from a range of problems, including poor educational achievement and emotional problems. The NSPCC identifies further problems, including:

- health hazards, like lack of food or clothing, carelessness or accidents;
- lack of parental supervision – forgetfulness or even unconsciousness;
- children dangerously copying their parents' behaviour;
- isolation of the family from neighbours and support services.

If you are caring for a child because the parent is a drug user, you are not alone. A 2011 survey of 255 grandparents by the support group Grandparents Plus found that almost half (46 per cent) were bringing up their grandchildren because the child's parent was addicted to drink or drugs.

Bringing up a child whose parents are drug addicts is not without its cost to wider family members. A study of 60 grandparents in the USA rearing children of drug-addicted parents found that although many found it emotionally rewarding, they also incurred psychological, physical and economic costs in performing their roles. You may lack the extra money that children inevitably need. You may feel that your parenting skills are rusty if you have grown-up children, and worry that you won't be able to meet a child's emotional needs. The child of a drug addict may have emotional and physical problems caused by the parent's addiction, which can mean that the child is more than usually difficult to care for. If this is a step that you are thinking about taking, make sure that you consider the wider impact to yourself and your family, and do as much as you can to put a support network in place. You will find many sources of help and advice in 'Useful addresses'.

A cousin's story

My cousin Karen had four children. She had been using drugs since she was a teenager. The first three children were taken into care and the fourth was adopted. I didn't find out that the three had been taken into care until months later, and I only found out that the fourth had been born at all – and subsequently adopted – until he was a year old. My family had been too embarrassed to tell anyone. Then when I contacted social services to ask about the fourth child, they told me that Karen had had a fifth, Adam. At the time, Karen was addicted to heroin and crack cocaine. Adam was also born addicted. He was taken from her at birth. She saw him for three days. She is currently missing and we don't know whether she is alive or dead.

When Adam was born it wasn't really a question of would we have him, as we'd already decided we would if she had any more. My partner was all for it – he was brought up in a large family and we'd already planned to adopt anyway. So it was lucky. There's been big issues with him coming because it is different, having a special guardianship order, the feeling's different from your own child. You get a lot of different things you have to deal with.

We didn't actually get him here until he was seven and a half months. It took four and a half months of assessment and interviews and medicals before he was allowed to come here. But in all that time we didn't actually see him. We were just told general snippets – he's fine, he's cut a tooth. You're not building any bond. They literally just turned up with him one day and said, 'Here you go.' He was seven and a half months old. He had problems. His foster mother hadn't put him in a sleep routine. She hadn't turned up for eye appointments even though he had a bad squint. He hadn't had a repeat brain scan after he had a cerebral haemorrhage at birth. He cried all the time. He'd obviously been affected by the moves he'd had. He'd been put into respite care before he came to us with a complete stranger. So it did take a while to get used to each other. It's not like having your own baby where you've carried them for nine months and you know them when they come out. We didn't know Adam at all.

He's much better now. He's got some cerebral palsy and he's probably going to be under the early programme support team. He doesn't walk as well as he should, he doesn't see as well as he should and his fine motor skills are not as good as they should be, and this is due to the drug taking. But he is doing better here, I think, than he would do in a foster home. I don't think even now he would have been adopted. They hadn't done a parallel plan. They had no clue where he was going if I hadn't turned up.

You don't get anything unless you scream and shout. I'm now an advocate for other mothers because they don't know what to say in meetings, they're completely railroaded. They are given residence orders, then are told you have to do this or that. If you've got a residence order, if it's not a child in need it's nothing to do with social services. You have to sit down with them and say these are your rights, this is what you should be saying. You don't need to be doing this. That's how we were when we got Adam. We were very demanding.

What's got me through is that I investigate everything. I never leave anything – I never trust anything that anyone in authority tells me unless I read it myself. I've found out that information is power. As soon as I found out that Adam was born I got in touch with the guardian, the social services – I never let them get a minute's peace. I was always on the phone demanding to know information, demanding to know his health and things like that.   (Carly)

A grandparent's story

My grandson is absolutely wonderful. In reality, the best thing that happened was him coming to us. He's got stability, he's got security, he's got love and affection. He's got nutrition. He's got everything that he needs. He fits in well with the community. He does all kinds of sports. He's a nice lad.

It was a hard decision. He was handed to me by a social worker. They said: 'Will you take him or shall we take him into care?' I said, 'Well, I'll take him for now and we'll sort it out.' I brought him back to our house. His maternal grandparents live locally. We assumed he would be going to them, being his mother's parents. We were happy about that as it's only down the road. The social worker came to see us the next day and said that social services had issues with the maternal grandmother and they would prefer him to come to us. So we were left with 24 hours to decide if he was going to us, if he was going to them, or if he would be taken into care. So we decided then that we would have him, in the hope that our son and their daughter would sort themselves out, be that a couple of years down the line or whatever. That they would sort themselves out and have him back. Of course, that hasn't been the case.

Obviously money comes into the equation. There was never any question about us having our grandson. Obviously we did. But I'm medically retired. I haven't got a great deal of money. I'm all right but not very well off. When I made inquiries to social services with regards to a residential order allowance, they told me, 'Oh no, this was a private arrangement, we have nothing to do with it' – even though the child was handed to me by a social worker. Then local services became involved, and they recommended that we apply for a residence order, which we did, with no mention of making an application for an allowance first. So they granted the residence order and washed their hands of it. We haven't seen them since.

It was a big decision. Eight years later, I know that we should have fought some more – I suppose we were looking at our son and their daughter through rose-coloured glasses, hoping that they would sort themselves out. Realistically, there wasn't much hope. But we were trying to do good by everyone. He was the priority – but also by our son and their daughter. But if it came to the choice between care and having him, then there is no choice – we would have him. Every grandparent would say the same.   (Alan)

If you want the children of a family member to live with you, you should get specialist advice as soon as possible. Family law is a complex area. The law is slightly different in England, Wales, Scotland and Northern Ireland, and is subject to change. Every case is different and you will find that there are several options open to you, each of which have their advantages and disadvantages. Several organizations provide help and advice for kinship carers – see 'Useful addresses' for more details.

Social services departments across the UK can vary wildly in terms of their attitudes and policies when it comes to finding care for children of drug addicts. Below, a helpline advisor offers his advice when dealing with social services:

- *The onus is on you to put yourself forward if you want to be considered as a carer.* It really depends on the social services department involved. I have spoken to many people where the local social services have gone straight to the grandparents when children have been removed from parents, and the children have been in the grandparents' care that night. I have also spoken to others who have been overlooked by social services and haven't had an assessment or anything like that and the children have been put into foster care, or up for adoption. So contact social services directly if you want to be considered.
- *Be prepared to deal with more than one social worker.* You could have three social workers in the space of three months. It's hard for grandparents to create a bond with a social worker when one comes round, talks to them, does an assessment, and the next time someone else comes round, and then another. These three different social workers might have three separate opinions. You might get on great with the first one and think things will be fine, the children will stay, and the second one will come and say, 'We don't want you to look after them.'
- *Be persistent.* Keep badgering on at social services. If you call them and someone says they'll get back to you, don't hold your breath. Keep calling.
- *Get everything in writing.* If a social worker ever says something like, 'We'd be happy for you to have the children', or 'We'd like

to give you financial assistance', get it in writing. If it's not in writing, they may back out of it.

- *Keep a paper trail.* From the moment you start, keep a diary, a scrapbook, anything like that, anything you can go back to. Keep notes of all calls made and when you made them.
- *Get advice before you start the process, if possible.* It's likely that you have never been in this situation before. So get in touch with the experts before you start the process. Your main concern will be getting the children, so you might agree to something straight away and then realize afterwards that your agreement includes various things that you might not have agreed if you'd known this or that. You do need to be cautious. Think of the children, but read through everything and speak to someone who knows what to do before you take action. For example, there is a residence order allowance paid by a local authority. But if it's not written in the court papers that the local authority will provide financial assistance, they will not pay it. They will say that it's not written in, so we're not going to pay it. This happens a lot. If the local authority agree to financial assistance, make sure it's written in before the actual residence order goes through.

5

Helping a family member with treatment

One of the first things on your mind when you discover that a family member is addicted to drugs will no doubt be: 'Can he be cured? And can I help him?'

It used to be thought that the family had no effect on whether or not the addict decided to seek treatment. However, over the last ten years, more research has been done which suggests that although a family member cannot control what an addict does, he or she may exert a positive influence. Many addicts cite family influence as a reason for entering treatment, and substance abuse services are being encouraged to involve family and social networks as much as possible when helping an addict make a decision about treatment.

So although every addict is different and every family is different – and with the familiar caveat that there is no single magic cure for drug addiction – it may well be that a family can make a difference. This chapter looks at the evidence that points to positive family influence, examines the different kinds of treatment options available in the UK, and discusses the main approaches that a family can take towards encouraging a drug user to enter treatment.

Can I make my family member seek treatment?

It's certainly true that only the user himself can make the ultimate decision to enter treatment – you can't force him to enter treatment against his will (although treatment may be a condition if the user is in the criminal justice system).

Studies have shown, however, that families can help influence an addict towards treatment, although much of the research in this area is focused on alcoholics and on specific kinds of treatments.

For example, one study asked the partners of drinkers to follow an approach known as 'Pressure to Change'. Briefly, this approach involves the family members putting pressure on the drinker – for example, rewarding the drinker for not drinking, taking part in activities which are incompatible with drinking, and working towards the 'Johnson Intervention' (see p. 70) as a last resort. This study found that two-thirds of those in treatment made a 'significant move' towards change.

Another US study offered 130 'significant others' of problem drinkers three different approaches to dealing with the problem drinker in the family – a 12-step programme, a 'confrontational family intervention' or the Community Reinforcement and Family Training (CRAFT) programme, which works with family members and uses techniques such as role-play and problem-solving. Thirteen per cent of the drinkers became involved in the 12-step programme, 30 per cent became involved in treatment after the intervention and 64 per cent became involved in treatment following the family training programme. The same researchers studied the effectiveness of the CRAFT programme with drug addicts. Three-quarters of the participants, who were taught various strategies, were able to engage the resistant family member in treatment during the six-month study period.

So it would appear that, whatever the approach available, engaging and involving the family of a drug user can be effective in getting the user to try and change. In fact, one study of opiate users found that three-quarters of the users cited family as their main reason for deciding to enter treatment.

There's also evidence to suggest that family influence doesn't just help the user go for treatment, it also helps him stay there and resist dropping out.

The addiction pathway

If you want to understand a little more about how an addiction can be broken, it's useful to think about the 'stages of change' model. This was developed by two psychologists, James Prochaska and Carlo DiClemente, and was originally applied to smokers. But it's since been applied to many other kinds of repeating behaviours, including drug and alcohol addiction.

Addiction isn't a disease which can be instantly 'cured'. Rather, according to the model, it's a process. Before we successfully overcome an addiction, we have to go through several stages. Everyone moves through those stages at their own rate and there's no set time for moving into and out of stages.

1 Pre-contemplation – the addict doesn't see any reason why he should change his behaviour. He believes that it's not impacting negatively on him or anyone around him.
2 Contemplation – the addict begins to realize that his behaviour is causing problems. But at this stage, he's not sure whether or not he wants to change.
3 Preparation – the addict has decided that he wants to change and starts getting ready. At this stage, for example, he might try to find out about treatment programmes in his area, or call a helpline.
4 Action – the addict is now making a real effort to change and may be in treatment.
5 Maintenance – the addict is keeping to his goals, not using drugs and attempting not to relapse.

Of course, the majority of human beings don't move smoothly between theoretical stages of change, and you shouldn't expect the user in your family to do so – you may even find that he can go backwards, wanting to change one day and refusing to admit that there is a problem the next. However, it can be useful to recognize your family member's behaviour within this pattern. Knowing which 'stage' he is at will help you respond appropriately. For example, an addict entering a stage of 'preparation', and actively seeking help and advice, may be more inclined to listen to you and accept your help in finding treatment than an addict who does not yet believe that he has a problem. Knowing that a former addict is now attempting to 'maintain' his new lifestyle will help you to encourage him, reward him and help him steer clear of triggers which could cause him to relapse – of which, more below.

Relapsing

'Relapse' is sometimes included as a sixth stage in the stages of change model. This is because drug addiction is recognized as a chronically relapsing condition: 40 to 60 per cent of drug addicts will relapse. It's something that you should expect if you have a drug user in your family.

However, there's a difference between a lapse – a temporary slip back into his old patterns – and a relapse. If the user has a lapse, he'll be able to pull himself up again quickly, get back on to his recovery plan and continue his new way of thinking. But if he has a relapse, he will slip back completely into his old ways of thinking and behaving, and may start the cycle all over again.

What causes relapse?

Everyone's triggers are different – everything from seeing friends to having a row could potentially cause a relapse – and it's impossible to tell how vulnerable a user is to a trigger at any particular time. But the following list might be useful if you're trying to understand why the user in your family has lapsed or relapsed:

- Negative emotions – the user experiences, for example, unhappiness, boredom, loneliness, depression, or anger caused by conflict.
- Pressure – the user reacts to direct pressure ('Go on, have a smoke, you'll feel better') or indirect pressure, such as just being around other people who are using a drug.
- Positive emotions – the user remembers how good it felt to take the drug and wants to feel that way again.
- Physical needs – the user feels that he needs the drug to stop withdrawal symptoms.

It's worth emphasizing again that relapse is something to be expected. Changing entrenched behaviours is hard, and few of us are able to do it instantly, with no slips. If the user in your family has a relapse, it may not be the end of his attempts to get clean. It may help for him to look back at what caused the relapse, to learn from his slip and try not to make the same mistake next time.

Different kinds of treatment

The kind of treatment available for drug users varies widely across the UK. Some areas will have better provision than others. Because of this variation, I have used the National Institute for Clinical Excellence (NICE) guidelines as a framework for giving you some idea of what might be available nationally (and what your area's services should be aiming for). In 2008, the government produced a report, *Protecting Families and Communities*, which stated that treatment services need to:

- work with families to get drug users into treatment;
- involve families and carers in planning treatment services;
- involve families in treatment;
- increase support and treatment for families;
- encourage families to stay together wherever possible;
- support kinship carers.

Finding out what's available in your area

Start with your local healthcare provider. Your GP should be able to tell you where to go next. A social worker will also have access to support service information, and if the user has had an emergency episode, A&E staff will also be able to advise you. You can also find your nearest substance abuse support team by calling FRANK, the national drugs helpline – see 'Useful addresses' for details.

Finding out what help is needed

If the user goes to a non-specialist first, such as a GP, he'll be asked various questions about his drug use. This is so that the GP, or social worker or probation officer, can assess how bad the problem is, how urgently help is needed, and where to send the drug user next.

The user is then likely to be referred to a specialist substance misuse service. Again, he will be assessed by the service, again being asked questions designed to work out how serious the problem is and what kind of help is needed. The user is also likely to be asked how motivated he is to enter treatment.

It may be that if the user's drug problem is very serious and there are other issues involved – such as mental health – he may be referred for a 'comprehensive assessment', which may involve more than one specialist health professional, such as a psychiatrist, or a doctor if the user needs prescription drugs such as methadone.

The user may be asked to take drugs tests during his assessments. For these tests, he will have to agree to give a urine or a saliva sample. He may need to give regular samples as he goes through the treatment process.

The aim of all these assessments is to come up with a care plan. This plan will be different for every drug user. Basically, it's an agreement between the user and his key worker on a plan of action, which will contain goals for the drug user to aim for. It should be short and easy to understand, and it should be the result of a collaboration between the user and his key worker. It should include details of treatment and any other areas of concern, such as housing, and it should be reviewed regularly.

The treatment plan may involve treatment in the community or residential treatment.

Questions to ask

A drug user doesn't have to tell his family that he is being treated for a drug problem, and medical staff have a duty of confidentiality to the person being treated. However, if you are involved in his treatment and care, NICE guidelines for England and Wales recommend that you should ask the following questions:

- Please give me some information about treatments for drug problems.
- Am I entitled to be told about the treatment my family member/ friend is having?
- What can we do to support the person with a drug problem?
- Can you give me any information about specialist support for families and carers, such as helplines and help during a crisis?

Community treatment

This kind of treatment is non-residential – hence the name. It might involve any of the following.

Prescription drugs

These are commonly prescribed to heroin users. The user will be prescribed a heroin substitute, either methadone or buprenorphine (brand name Subutex). The idea behind substitute prescribing is to provide an alternative to heroin, which the user will not have to pay for, thus lessening the risk that he will commit a crime to pay for his heroin. The substitute will be taken by mouth, thus reducing the risks associated with injecting. It will also stave off withdrawal symptoms, allowing the user instead to cut down gradually if that is what he wants. The substitute will be prescribed either by a GP or by a specialist substance abuse support team.

If you are living with a user who is taking a prescribed heroin substitute, remember that these are still dangerous and extremely powerful drugs. Methadone in particular is very easy to overdose on, particularly if the person taking the drug has not taken it before. A dose which has little effect on a regular user may be enough to kill someone with no tolerance. Consequently, the methadone must be kept in a very safe place which cannot be accessed by children. There have been several tragic cases where children of drug addicts have died after ingesting methadone, either given to them by their parents to make them sleep or consumed by accident. All methadone must be dispensed in a childproof container. To reduce these risks, the user may be asked to attend a treatment centre or go to a pharmacy daily to take his dose.

The user may then decide to gradually reduce his dose in order to wean himself slowly off his addiction. This should be done in consultation with his key worker and doctor if necessary.

Counselling

Counselling will help the user talk through how he feels, and take into account any underlying problems which might influence his decision to use drugs.

Support groups

These may be provided by local support services, or by a programme such as those run by Narcotics Anonymous.

Residential treatment

This option involves going into hospital or a residential rehabilitation centre.

Inpatient treatment

Withdrawing from any drug can involve very unpleasant side effects and can be dangerous to undergo without medical supervision. Detoxing in hospital means that the user will be given other drugs and medical help to make the detox easier to deal with. If he has any other health problems, these can also be dealt with in a hospital.

Where is inpatient treatment available?

A user can access inpatient treatment in the psychiatric ward of a general hospital, in a specialist drug unit within a hospital, or in the detox unit of a residential rehabilitation centre. Provision of these services is patchy and what's available to the user depends on where he is in the UK. Your local substance abuse team should be able to tell you what kind of treatment is available, where it is and what the drug user needs to do in order to access it – he may need to be referred to the unit by the local substance abuse team.

Residential rehab

This takes place in residential centres where the user will be expected to stay for a considerable period. Some rehabs have programmes lasting for weeks, others for months. They vary widely in their approaches and may involve:

* individual talking therapy;
* group therapy;
* workshops;

- development of coping strategies for when the programme ends;
- family therapy;
- activities such as swimming, exercise and art therapy;
- aftercare programmes and meetings for those who have gone through a residential rehab programme.

The majority of residential centres require the user to go through a detox programme before he starts the residential programme, which could be done at another hospital or at the centre itself. The user will be asked to abide by a list of residential rules, and most will make it a condition of stay that no drugs are to be used. If the rules are broken, the user may be asked to leave.

The cost of residential rehab varies depending on the provider, but it is not cheap. However, it is possible to be referred to residential rehab via the NHS, but again this depends on where you live and what services are available, and there is likely to be a long waiting list. Some medical insurance packages will fund residential rehab, so if you have this it's worth checking to see what is covered.

Some treatment phrases you may encounter

'Tough love'

Crudely, this is the concept of 'being cruel to be kind'. For example, if you refuse to give your family member money to buy drugs even though he is suffering withdrawal symptoms, that could be seen as 'tough love' – the decision is made out of a genuine desire to help the addict, not a desire to see him suffer. It's a wide concept now used to describe everything from the above situation to not allowing your children to eat as many sweets as they like, and is touted as a cure for everything from juvenile delinquency to obesity.

Again, how useful this idea is to your own situation is up to you. There is no consensus as to just how effective 'tough love' really is, and no conclusive research. However, there's no doubt that taking any kind of drastic step – for example, telling the user he must leave the family home, or withdrawing financial support – must be considered very carefully, as it can backfire.

'Rock bottom'

This is a pleasingly dramatic phrase, so it can frequently be found in newspapers and magazines describing how a certain actress, singer or all-round celebrity hit an all-time mental, physical and spiritual low. It describes the point in an addict's life where he can go no lower. It's supposed to be at this point that the addict is more amenable to change. Hence, the families of addicts are sometimes urged to allow the user to 'hit rock bottom' – the theory runs that the family should not intervene, as the sooner the addict hits this point, the sooner he will seek help.

Again, this may be a useful concept to you, but before applying it you may want to consider:

- Can I help the user to change? Have I done everything in my power to help him change?
- How far am I prepared to allow the user to go before I intervene?
- What are the consequences of allowing him to hit 'rock bottom'? What effect will they have, not just on him but also on me and my family?
- Will the user actually seek change as a consequence of hitting 'rock bottom'?

Should I try and make him stop at home?

A user doesn't necessarily need to enter treatment in order to get off his drug of choice, or start taking a substitute such as methadone. It is possible for him to withdraw simply by stopping the drug – a 'home detox', during which the user will go through withdrawal, or 'cold turkey'. He may ask you to help him with this, or you may decide to try and persuade him to do it. Sometimes it is done as a last resort when all else has failed, and sometimes it's for other reasons – such as a drug user who wants to quit but doesn't want to talk to any kind of medical professional, perhaps because he is wanted by the police.

If this is a road you would like to go down, always speak to a medical professional before you start. Withdrawal symptoms, both psychological and physical, vary depending on the drug of choice and can be extremely upsetting to witness. The user may also become violent or aggressive, or plead with you to let him go. A home detox is likely to be a painful experience for you and the user, and you will need to prepare yourself. Stopping any drug use suddenly can also be dangerous – for example, stopping benzodiazepines and barbiturates suddenly can cause seizures, which can be fatal. Going 'cold turkey' with alcohol can result in serious cases of *delirium tremens*, which can again be fatal. If the user is taking any of these drugs, or is also addicted to alcohol, he should always be under the care of a medical professional if he decides to withdraw.

Different kinds of intervention

If you've been on the internet to research possible ways of helping the drug user in your family, you will no doubt have come across the concept of intervention. This term can be used to describe anything from a chat with a health professional about the user's drug use to a full-scale planned confrontation involving the family, friends and a professional counsellor or 'interventionist'.

Brief interventions

Studies have shown that brief interventions by health professionals can be effective for people whose drug use hasn't yet reached 'serious' levels. For those with a more serious problem, they can help encourage the user to enter a more specialized treatment programme, or refer him to other services which can provide help. A brief intervention would typically take the form of the health professional helping the user to identify what stage of harm his substance use has reached and the costs and benefits of continuing to use the substance, and discussing strategies to help the user cut down – the kind of intervention discussed in the section on community treatment on p. 65. It's very different from a so-called 'orchestrated' intervention by the family, as we shall see.

'Psychosocial' interventions

This is a phrase used to describe a range of services designed to help the user give up. It might involve psychological treatments such as cognitive behavioural therapy or counselling, or a 'rewards' or 'incentives' programme, where the user is given a reward if a drug test shows that he is drug-free.

'Orchestrated' interventions

An orchestrated or planned intervention is done without the prior knowledge or consent of the user. Family and friends, with the help of a professional counsellor, get together to 'stage' an intervention, which is carefully planned in advance. Family and friends are encouraged to write letters, telling the user how his behaviour is affecting them and listing rules that he must follow and the consequences of not following these rules. Telling the user that he must enter treatment or face expulsion from the home, or another serious consequence, is common. The user will then be unexpectedly confronted by the concerned group. The group read out their letters and the user must then make his decision.

Does it work? There is no doubt that some families find orchestrated interventions effective. One particular advantage from the family's point of view is that they are encouraged to play an active role in seeking treatment for the family member's problem, and in many cases an intervention programme will also include counselling and support for the family. This can be a very attractive proposition for families who feel that previous attempts at getting help for the user have just involved counselling and support for the user and not for his family.

However, there are concerns about just how effective these interventions can be in the long term, and research is inconclusive. The 'Johnson Intervention' is probably the best-known intervention programme, adhering to the method described above, and evidence as to its effectiveness is mixed. A 1999 evaluation of the Johnson Method studied 24 families of alcoholics. Out of these, only seven went through with the final evaluation, suggesting that deciding to go through with an intervention is viewed as a very drastic step.

The research also found that those alcoholics who were 'confronted' were more likely to enter treatment.

However, the long-term effectiveness of the Johnson Method has been called into question. Another study of the Johnson Method found high relapse rates and noted: 'Although individuals who undergo a Johnson Intervention are most likely to enter treatment, the power of the Johnson Intervention to retain clients deteriorates over the course of treatment, as indicated by their diminished likelihood of completing.'

This kind of intervention is generally expensive. It goes without saying that before considering it you should thoroughly research the intervention provider. You may want to consider the following questions:

- Exactly what form will the intervention take?
- What will be required of me and my family?
- How will you support and prepare us?
- What is your long-term success rate? Do you have records for how many of your clients relapse within the year?
- What kind of addictions do your other clients suffer from – are you experienced in the particular addiction that my family member is going through?
- What kind of follow-up support is available for the user and for the family?
- What experience and qualifications do your staff have?
- What happens if the intervention fails?

Helping your family member through treatment

So evidence suggests that family members can help guide users towards treatment, keep them going once they are there, and play a part in preventing relapse after they leave. But how should you support your family member through this process?

- Be there with information when he needs it. Find out about all the options available locally. You do not have to be a drug user to access substance abuse support services – they should be ready and willing to give a family member all the information needed. Talk to the user about making changes and practical ways in which he might go about making these changes.

- Get support for yourself. As has been previously discussed, your own wellbeing and that of your family is just as important as the wellbeing of the addict. Being able to discuss your situation with others who are going through the same thing, or with substance abuse professionals, will help you to see your own situation more clearly.
- Support any positive changes in the user's behaviour. Use rewards, but only when the user has stopped using drugs.
- Learn to recognize triggers in the user's pattern of drug use and plan for them accordingly. For example, you might want to help the user stay away from a social circle who use drugs.
- Remember that relapse is a part of addiction. Getting clean from drugs can take a long time. Again, it's worth emphasizing that there is no magic bullet to 'cure' drug addiction. If the user relapses, this isn't necessarily the end of the recovery process. If you feel that helping the user start treatment again would be positive, carry on supporting him and encouraging him to go back and start again.

6

Drugs of addiction – a brief guide

The world of drugs is changing all the time. Some drugs fall out of fashion and aren't widely used. Some, like heroin and cocaine, seem to have been around for ever. New forms of old drugs, such as crack, appear as if out of nowhere and suddenly become widely available. Some rise and fall with a certain 'scene', such as LSD and the hippies in the 1960s, or ecstasy and the rave scene in the late 1980s and early 1990s. And over the last few years, entirely new drugs like mephedrone have surfaced – cheap, easy to manufacture, very profitable to sell over the internet and, until the government was informed of its existence, entirely legal. So it may well be that by the time you are reading this, the drug landscape has changed once again.

The purpose of this chapter is to give a brief rundown of the major drugs of abuse and their effects. You may already know plenty about the drug your family member is abusing. However, the drug world is a closed one. It has its own language, its own etiquette and its own rules. If you're not a drug user and you don't work in a relevant field, it's unlikely that you will have come into contact with it before. Knowledge is power. Knowing a little about the drugs themselves, their effects, how users refer to them and how much they cost will help demystify this world in which your family member seems so at ease, and in which you feel like an outsider.

> My parents were sort of really clean living when they grew up so I think it was a shock for them when my brother started to encounter those issues [with drugs]. They were unprepared for it and I think that's why they just didn't know what to do. They couldn't sit him down and say, 'Look, son, we've all been there when we're 17' – they hadn't gone through that stuff and neither have I, as my brother's experience turned me right off that stuff. (Lisa)

My parents knew nothing about drugs but they learned very, very fast once they knew my brother had a problem. My mum became something of an expert. I think it helped her, actually, doing the research, it made her feel that there was something positive she could do.   (Marcus)

Each of the drugs described here comes with the same caveat – there is no way to know exactly how much of the actual substance is present in what's being taken. Purity varies widely and drugs can also be 'cut' with various other potentially harmful substances to bulk them out.

Prices can only ever be approximate as these change depending on the availability of the drug and where in the UK the drug is being sold.

Using more than one drug (polydrug use)

It is common for a drug addict to use more than one drug. Indeed, one study points out that if alcohol and cigarettes are included, most drug users are polydrug users. Combinations of drugs are used for several reasons – to enhance the effects (such as 'speedballing' – taking a mixture of heroin and cocaine), to combat the effects of one drug by using another (for example, using tranquillizers to get to sleep after using a stimulant such as cocaine or speed) or simply because the drugs in question are the only ones available. Naturally, the risk of overdose or other adverse effects becomes higher with every drug used.

This book doesn't examine alcohol abuse, but it's worth noting that one of the commonest forms of drug mixing occurs with a drug plus alcohol. This is also one of the most dangerous ways of mixing drugs, particularly with opiates, cocaine and tranquillizers.

The following drug pairings are particularly risky:

- Mixing alcohol and cocaine increases the user's risk of cardiovascular toxicity (damage to the heart). The combination results in the liver producing a compound called cocaethylene, which, it is believed, increases the risk of a heart attack.

- Mixing alcohol and/or depressant drugs with opiates increases the risk of overdose.
- Mixing alcohol and benzodiazepines can lead to mood changes, such as increased aggression.
- Mixing cannabis and cocaine can increase the user's heart rate above levels which are the norm for just using either one of the drugs by itself, increasing the risk of a heart attack.

The UK's major drugs of addiction

Amphetamines

What it's called, what it looks like and how much it costs

Amphetamine (speed, whizz) comes in powder form of varying colours – brown, pink and white are common. It costs around £9 per gram.

How is it taken?

It's snorted, swallowed or sometimes injected.

What does it do?

It's a stimulant, so it gives the user a huge amount of energy. Taking amphetamines is popular with clubbers as it enables them to dance for long periods of time without getting tired.

Like cocaine, amphetamines put a strain on the heart, putting users at a higher risk of stroke or a heart attack. They keep the user awake, so he might suffer from lack of sleep along with the other physical effects, or use other drugs in order to get to sleep. Amphetamines suppress the appetite – they were used legally as a diet drug by many women in the 1950s and 1960s – and using them regularly can result in paranoia and anxiety attacks.

Legal status

In powder form, speed is a Class B drug, while speed prepared for injection is a Class A drug. Possession can result in a prison sentence of up to five years. Supplying the drug can mean an unlimited fine and up to 14 years in jail.

Cannabis

What it's called, what it looks like and how much it costs

Cannabis (green, blow, skunk, weed, dope) is sold either as herbal cannabis – green buds and leaves – or as 'hash' or 'soapbar', which usually looks like a sticky brown-black lump similar to liquorice in appearance. This is made from the plant's resin. Hash costs around £50 per ounce, while herbal cannabis costs between £90 and £130 for an ounce. Again, how much a person gets through depends on how addicted he is. A heavy user might get through as much as an ounce a week. It's usually sold in small plastic bags and can have a strong herbal smell. It's the most commonly used illegal drug in the UK.

> My brother hit adolescence and starting experimenting with cannabis mainly, but I know he got caught by my parents sniffing aerosols and stuff like that with his mates. Once he hit 13 or 14 he didn't ever really get out of that cycle of substance misuse. By the time he was in his early 20s he was a real heavy cannabis user and I know that he tried literally everything else. I know that he's done ecstasy and he had tried heroin and cocaine but he never developed problems with those.   (Lisa)

How is it taken?

It's usually crumbled into 'joints' – hand-rolled cigarettes – and mixed with tobacco. It can also be smoked through a pipe (a 'bong'), heated on a knife with the smoke being inhaled ('hot knives') or put into food like cookies or cakes.

What does it do?

Cannabis usually has a relaxing effect, with users becoming happy, giggly and slightly detached. They may feel hungry ('getting the munchies') or experience mild hallucinatory effects such as becoming more aware of colours, textures and sounds. However, some also report paranoia and nausea. Smoking also damages the heart and lungs. It is certainly possible to become addicted to cannabis, although the substance doesn't have the same addictive qualities as heroin or cocaine.

You may have heard about reports linking cannabis use to an increased risk of developing schizophrenia. But the link is still not clear. It certainly seems to be the case that many schizophrenics and people with other mental illnesses report using cannabis. What's not known is whether these people were already at higher risk of mental illness before they started using cannabis. Some scientists believe that cannabis could somehow 'trigger' an underlying mental illness, though the exact process behind this is also not yet known.

Legal status

Cannabis is a Class B drug. Possession can result in a prison sentence of up to five years. Supplying the drug can mean an unlimited fine and up to 14 years in jail.

Cocaine and crack cocaine

What it's called, what it looks like and how much it costs

Cocaine (coke, charlie, toot, C) is a white powder. It usually comes in a paper wrap or a small plastic bag. It costs around £40 for a gram of cocaine and £10 for a 'rock' of crack (also known as freebase or base). How much an addict uses depends on how addicted he is, but as the effects of both drugs wear off quite quickly it's not unknown for an addict to use several grams in a weekend, or a few rocks in a day.

How is it taken?

Cocaine is commonly snorted through a rolled-up piece of paper or banknote but can also be injected. Crack cocaine is usually smoked through a pipe, which could be a glass tube, a bottle, a foil pipe or even an empty drink can.

What does it do?

Users report that cocaine gives a great boost to energy and confidence. They feel invincible and wide awake. However, these effects wear off quickly, meaning the user has to take more in a short period of time.

Repeated use can also result in paranoia and aggression, insomnia, and physical damage to the nose if the drug is being snorted and to the lungs if it's being smoked. Injecting is extremely dangerous. The addict has no way of knowing how much active ingredient is in the solution he is injecting. He also has no way of knowing how strong it is, and once it is in the bloodstream it can't be taken out. Therefore, the danger of overdose is significant. Sharing needles can spread HIV or other blood-borne diseases such as hepatitis C. According to the Department of Health, 90 per cent of all cases of hepatitis C and 6 per cent of all HIV cases in England are caused by injecting drugs. Injection sites can easily become infected and long-term injecting can cause the user's veins to collapse.

Cocaine and crack are stimulants and cause the heart to beat faster, increasing the risks of a heart attack. It's very risky to take either if you have heart problems or high blood pressure. Taking cocaine or crack along with other drugs, including alcohol, increases the risk of side effects. They are both highly addictive substances.

Legal status

Like heroin, cocaine and crack cocaine are Class A substances under the Misuse of Drugs Act. Possessing or supplying them can result in a prison sentence or a fine. Possession can lead to a prison sentence of up to seven years and an unlimited fine, while supplying could result in a life sentence.

Ecstasy

What it's called, what it looks like and how much it costs

Ecstasy (pills, tabs, Es, doves, Mandy) is the common name for pills containing the chemical MDMA. Pills can come in any colour – white, white with brown specks, blue, pink and brown are common – and will usually be stamped with a logo. The pill is also referred to by the logo – for example, a pill with a dove logo will be a 'dove'. Pills are usually sold in small plastic bags. In recent years, MDMA 'crystal' has appeared. This substance is a grey-white powder containing crystals, usually sold in a paper wrap. A pill costs around £3.

How is it taken?

Pills are usually swallowed, though they can also be crushed, then snorted or crumbled into roll-up cigarettes and smoked. MDMA crystal can be rubbed on to the gums or wrapped in paper and swallowed ('bombed').

What does it do?

Ecstasy users will experience a 'rush' of pleasure when the drug takes effect. This is then followed by a sense of well-being, calmness, happiness and empathy, plus the urge to dance. They may chew or grin compulsively, have dilated pupils, be 'twitchy' or be unable to complete a coherent sentence.

When they are 'coming down' and the effect of the drug is wearing off, they may have problems sleeping. Users commonly report feeling depressed and down a few days after taking the drug – the 'midweek blues'. It can raise the body temperature to very high levels, causing heatstroke. Drinking some water to avoid dehydration is advised, but not too much. The most well-known ecstasy death, that of Leah Betts, was caused by 'water intoxication' – drinking too much water in an attempt to avoid dehydration.

How addictive ecstasy is has long been debated. Users certainly report taking large amounts and needing to take more in order to achieve the desired effect. However, it doesn't seem to set off a similar compulsion to that of heroin, crack or cocaine.

Legal status

It's a Class A drug. Possession can lead to a prison sentence of up to seven years and an unlimited fine, while supplying could result in a life sentence.

GHB/GBL

What it's called, what it looks like and how much it costs

GHB (gammahydroxybutrate) and GBL (gammabutyrolactone) are also known as 'liquid ecstasy'. GHB and GBL are similar drugs from the same family. They are not related to ecstasy, however, despite the nickname. They can be very hard to tell apart and have very similar effects. Once GBL is ingested, it converts to GHB in the user's body.

GHB is usually sold in bottles as a clear, odourless liquid, though it is also available in powder form. GBL is also a clear liquid, but it has a slight chemical smell. It's a solvent, commonly used in paint stripper. A small bottle of GHB or GBL costs around £15, though it's also available in 'capfuls'.

How is it taken?

It's taken orally in 'doses' measured in either millilitres or capfuls.

What does it do?

GHB and GBL are often taken as substitutes for alcohol. They relax the user and give a sense of well-being and sleepiness. Other side effects include nausea and dizziness, plus depression and exhaustion in the days following a GHB/GBL dose.

It's worth mentioning that GHB and GBL are extremely dangerous as they are very easy to overdose on. There's no consensus as to what the standard 'dose' should be and no way of knowing how concentrated the substance is. When other drugs, especially alcohol, are taken at the same time, the dangers increase. Just a small amount can lead to vomiting, unconsciousness and death even in regular users. It is possible to become addicted to GHB and GBL.

Legal status

Both GHB and GBL are Class C drugs. Possession can result in an unlimited fine and up to two years in prison. Supplying can result in an unlimited fine and a prison sentence of up to 14 years.

Heroin

What it's called, what it looks like and how much it costs

Heroin is also known as smack, skag, gear, brown, China White, junk, horse or H. It usually comes in the form of a white or brown powder, most commonly stored in a small paper 'wrap'. A DrugLink survey in 2005 found the street price of a gram to be £50. The average addict needs a quarter to half a gram every day. Methadone (not to be confused with mephedrone, a completely different drug) is a heroin substitute commonly legally prescribed to heroin addicts who are trying to kick the habit, but it is also sold illegally to heroin addicts. It usually takes the form of a dark-green liquid which is taken by mouth.

How is it taken?

It can be snorted, smoked ('chasing the dragon') or injected ('shooting up'). It's a member of the opiate class of drugs, and one of the most addictive illegal drugs. Users may start off by smoking the drug; then, as they become more addicted and develop a tolerance, they begin injecting for the almost instantaneous effect this gives.

Heroin is prepared for injection by 'cooking' it in a spoon over a lighter, which produces a liquid that can then be injected. It is usually smoked in foil, with the user holding a lighter under the foil to heat the heroin and using a self-rolled foil pipe to inhale. Burned or missing spoons and burned foil may be signs that someone in your household is using heroin. Injecting heroin also carries all the risks noted in the 'Cocaine' section (see p. 78).

What does it do to the body?

Opiates have been popular for centuries with recreational users, and the reason behind that is their pleasurable effects. Heroin produces a feeling of intense well-being to the exclusion of all else. Users have spoken of feeling totally detached from any problems they might have, of a comforting 'wall' between themselves and reality. As tolerance develops, this effect becomes less pronounced and the addict will find himself taking more and more simply to feel normal.

Heroin has other physical effects. It can make the user very sick, though this usually stops or lessens after the first few hits. It dilates the pupils. The user will seem 'dopey', detached and inattentive, sleepy and relaxed, 'nodding out'. He may scratch himself a lot, as opiates can cause itching. Too much, and the user will go into a coma and may even die from respiratory failure.

Heroin's intensely addictive nature means that addicts will very quickly find themselves desperate for money to buy it. This usually means that they turn to crime. Family members are the easiest targets for initial theft, and therefore vanishing cash and electrical goods may be an early sign that all is not well. This addictive nature also means that a heroin addiction is hard to treat successfully. An attempt to assess the combined harm caused by various drugs – including their potential to harm the body, induce dependence and damage the wider societal framework – found that heroin was top of the list.

Legal status

Under the Misuse of Drugs Act, heroin is a Class A substance. That means possessing it or supplying it can result in a prison sentence or a fine. Possession can lead to a prison sentence of up to seven years and an unlimited fine, while supplying could result in a life sentence. In the eyes of the law, giving heroin to a friend is counted as 'supplying'.

Ketamine

What it's called, what it looks like and how much it costs

Ketamine (K, Special K, Vitamin K, ket) usually comes as a pill, a white powder or white crystals and is also available in liquid form. If it's a liquid, it will be 'cooked' (heated) to produce a powder. The powder is usually snorted while pills are swallowed. It can also be injected. It costs around £20 for a gram.

What does it do?

Ketamine is used legally as an anaesthetic on both humans and animals. Its effects can be very powerful. Users report feeling totally detached from themselves and their surroundings, and may hallucinate or experience strange out-of-body sensations, known as 'going down the K-hole'. Familiar objects or people may look totally different. The user may appear completely oblivious of his actual surroundings and be unable to communicate. Nausea is also common and high doses can knock a person out completely or even cause death – asphyxiation from inhaling vomit while unconscious is a particular risk. As ketamine is a depressant, it can affect breathing and the heart. Recent research has found a link between regular ketamine use and bladder and kidney damage.

Legal status

Ketamine is a Class C drug. Possession can result in an unlimited fine and up to two years in prison. Supplying can result in an unlimited fine and a prison sentence of up to 14 years.

Mephedrone/cathinones

Mephedrone (m-cat, meow meow, meph, drone) is a white powder. It was legally sold over the internet before being banned along with all other cathinones (see below) in April 2010. Many sites labelled it 'plant food – not for human consumption' to get around legislation, but it is not plant food and never has been. It belongs to a family of drugs called cathinones, which are similar to amphetamines. Other similar cathinone drugs were also sold over the internet prior to the ban, including methylone. It cost between £10 and £15 for a gram before the ban but it's not known how the price may have changed since then.

What does it do?

Its effects are similar to those of speed and ecstasy. The user will feel stimulated, excited, talkative and happy, and will have lots of energy. Because the drug is so new, there's very little reliable evidence available about what its dangers might be. Anecdotal evidence from users suggests that side effects include vasoconstriction – with parts of the body such as knees and fingertips turning purple – nausea, paranoia, increased heart rate and blackouts. Users have also reported a strong need to keep taking the drug until it's all gone. Snorting large amounts of the drug can damage the nose and throat. Anecdotally, it certainly seems to have addictive properties, though more research is needed.

Legal status

It's a Class B drug. Possession can result in a prison sentence of up to five years. Supplying the drug can mean an unlimited fine and up to 14 years in jail.

Methamphetamine

What it's called, what it looks like and how much it costs

Methamphetamine (crystal meth, yaba, ice, crank) is a form of amphetamine which is sold as a white or yellow powder or in small 'chips' – hence the nickname 'ice'. It can be smoked, snorted or injected. It costs between £35 and £75 for a gram.

What does it do?

The effects are similar to those of speed, but much stronger. Users experience a rush of energy and exhilaration. The risks as well as the effects are also increased. The drug puts a massive strain on the heart. It suppresses the appetite and keeps the user awake for long periods. It can also affect the mind, with users reporting psychosis, delusions, paranoia and violent behaviour. Methamphetamine is highly addictive and users can develop a tolerance very quickly, meaning that they will need to take more and more to get the desired effect.

Legal status

Methamphetamine is a Class A drug.

Solvents

What they're called, what they look like and how much they cost

Unlike the street drugs detailed in this chapter, you're likely to have plenty of solvents in your house already. They are chemicals present in a wide range of household goods, including aerosols like air fresheners, hairsprays and household cleaners. Solvents are also present in some computer keyboard dust remover sprays, lighter fuel, glues and paints, paint thinners and correction fluid. They are all widely available for a few pounds.

What do they do?

Solvents are commonly inhaled ('huffed') from a cloth, a plastic bag or even a sleeve. Gas products are squirted down the throat. The effect is similar to being drunk, with feelings of euphoria, nausea and dizziness being reported. The 'high' doesn't last long, so many users will repeat the dose within a short space of time, resulting in overdose.

Using solvents in this way is extremely dangerous. In particular, squirting gas down the throat can cause swelling, meaning that the person won't be able to breathe. They have been known to cause fatal heart failure on a first dose. Long-term use can cause brain, liver and kidney damage. There is no way to know how much is too much, and there is no such thing as safe use of solvents. Solvent abuse is very common in young people in particular. A fifth of people aged 15 to 16 in the UK have tried solvents and it is possible to become addicted to them.

Legal status

It's illegal for UK shopkeepers to sell gas lighter refills to anyone under 18. The law on solvents varies slightly in England and Scotland: in England, it's illegal for shopkeepers to sell 'intoxicating substances' to people under 18 who they think will misuse them. In Scotland, if a shopkeeper sells a substance 'recklessly' to anyone he or she thinks will misuse it – no matter what their age – prosecution can result.

Tranquillizers

What they're called, what they look like and how much they cost

Tranquillizers (bennies, uppers, downers, roofies, vallies, jellies) are drugs which are legally prescribed for conditions such as anxiety and depression. There are many different kinds, all with slightly different effects. It's not possible to give details of every single one here, so I have concentrated on the ones most commonly abused. They usually come in tablet form, in many different shapes and colours. They are sold either by street dealers or over the internet, at wildly varying prices. They are usually diverted from legitimate sources, such as stolen from hospitals or sold by addicts who have been prescribed them. A Royal Pharmaceutical Society survey carried out in 2009 estimated that up to 50 per cent of drugs sold over the internet will be counterfeit.

Some of the most commonly abused tranquillizers include diazepam (Valium), temazepam and lorazepam (Ativan). These are part of the benzodiazepine drug family. Non-benzodiazepines which are abused include zaleplon, zolpidem and zopiclone (the Z-drugs.)

Users have been known to crumble up tablets and inject them. While all injecting is highly dangerous, injecting in this form is even more so, as tablets contain chalk which can severely damage veins, leading to amputation.

What do they do?

Tranquillizers make the user feel relaxed and free of tension. They are commonly used in combination with other 'party' drugs such as speed and ecstasy in order to help the user 'come down' and relax. Used in conjunction with other drugs, and especially alcohol, they can be very dangerous, as this can lead to a fatal overdose. They are addictive and users can build up a high tolerance and need to use more to get an effect. Coming off benzodiazepines suddenly can cause very serious symptoms, including convulsions and acute anxiety. It's recommended that a long-term user of these drugs should only withdraw under medical supervision.

Legal status

Tranquillizers are only legal if you have been prescribed them. They are Class C drugs, which means that possession can lead to a prison sentence of up to two years. Supplying tranquillizers could result in a prison sentence of up to 14 years, plus an unlimited fine.

7

Afterword

A family is a complex entity, as is addiction. Dealing with this addiction within the family is a highly personal process, as every family and every addiction is different. Some stories end happily, others less so, and nobody can predict how your particular story will pan out.

Some things, however, we can say with some certainty. We know that learning about your family member's addiction and different ways in which he might overcome this addiction is helpful. We know that it's helpful for carers of drug addicts to take steps to safeguard their own mental and physical health, and to seek support in dealing with the situation. We know that families can encourage users to seek treatment, and can help them stay clean after treatment has finished. We know that treatment can be effective, but we also know that a family has every right to decide that it can no longer support a drug user. And we know that despite experiencing the trauma of a drug user within the family, families can survive.

Whatever your situation, I hope that this book has provided you with, if not definitive answers, some ideas as to how you might start your journey with a drug user in the family, or some indication as to a new direction that journey might take.

My brother has now been clean for five years. He's got his own flat. He's not really settled with a job yet but he's getting there. I don't know whether it's his own personality or the fact that we put up with his situation that has helped. I know that it's been a very long road for him, and for my parents. I think that it's really a combination of that initial impetus to get clean and his own determination to sort out his personal problems. Since he got clean, he's been in counselling. I think he really wanted to know the reason why he got addicted in the first place and the therapy has really helped him develop a positive self-image. He still gets depressed from time to time but as far as I know he hasn't gone back to the drugs.

(Marcus)

He's still around. He's not welcome here any more. That was last August – the final straw. He came in and stole documentation that resulted in him defrauding us of £15,000. I haven't personally spoken to him since. You live with it on a daily basis. For example, it was on the news this morning that a car had crashed in a local town. An event that happens a thousand times a day. But we immediately think: is that him? I just picked up the local paper now and it said that police had arrested a 35-year-old with a large quantity of amphetamines. Immediately you think: is that David? So it's with you constantly. I'm waiting for a knock on the door to say that they found him dead. I don't mean to be cold about it but that is how things have progressed. You know full well that that is the only outcome. It's not a question of will it, it's a question of when. That's how we feel.

(Alan)

I will have to take responsibility for my brother eventually. I could understand if someone said, 'You're not his parent, you don't have to assume that responsibility.' I can understand that perspective, but it feels like he's got nobody. That would be cruel, to not see yourself as having some responsibility to someone, when at that point you might be the only person they really have in the world. I think I've always felt that there would be a lot of stuff to deal with in the future when I'm older and when my parents aren't around. I wouldn't rule out any help in the future. I think it will probably get harder the older we get.

(Lisa)

To be honest, I resent him. I hate him for what he's done to his son. I still love him. He's still my son. But my priority is his son. He has contact with him every other Saturday. He has to ring me up to confirm and arrange times on a Friday. He's done that every time. That's the only contact I have with Steve. I haven't let myself get involved with his life. I don't know what he does. He could be off his head for the other 13 days but as long as he has shown concern to his son – he's my priority, that little boy. I don't trust Steve. When he takes his son swimming, I'm always looking for needle marks. While he hasn't stolen for years, I would not trust him. If he does start doing training, gets a job, has a life, that might come. But there are a lot of bridges to build. For all his good intentions, since he came out of prison, he's now on Incapacity Benefit because you get more money. But in the seven months he's been out, he hasn't been in any trouble. He is doing well. Hopefully he's turned a corner, but time will tell.

(Miriam)

Karen has now disappeared. Nobody knows where she is. I've asked social services if they do find her, can they please phone me and I will go to the hospital and I am going to talk to her about having a contraceptive implant. I would be the first member of my family to talk to her for about four years. She hates my uncle [Karen's father] now. Once he stopped giving her money, she just stopped getting in contact. So now I feel that one of us needs to go down there and speak to her and it'll be down to me. I wouldn't ever wish any harm to happen to her. But I'm quite hardened to her. I wouldn't like her to appear in our lives now. I think she would do nothing but damage to Adam. But the very fact that she abandoned every one of her children – she has no contact with any of them – is a comfort to me in a way. I'm in a very lucky position. I don't have to put up with her coming round once a month, drunk or off her face. I don't have to worry about Adam being open to that. But I do worry about her and I know that pretty soon I'll get another phone call and it will say that she's either dead or had another baby. And I know that I'll be the first port of call for the next baby because they've told me they will call me, and I'm going to have to make one of the most difficult decisions of my life. Whether to say yes or no. And I still from day to day don't know what I'll say.

(Carly)

Useful addresses

Provision of support services across the UK varies enormously and is constantly changing. It's also likely that changes in the structure of the NHS will affect these services in the near future. For this reason I haven't listed individual support groups or local service providers, but have concentrated on national organizations whose members are in touch with service providers on the ground and will be able to point you towards what's available in your area.

Support for families

Action on Addiction
Head Office
East Knoyle
Salisbury
Wilts SP3 6BE
Helpline: 0845 126 4130
Website: www.actiononaddiction.org.uk
Offers support groups for families, partners and friends of substance misusers, counselling and a brief residential programme (the Family Programme) for friends and relatives. There are linked offices in other parts of England.

Addaction
Central Office
67–69 Cowcross Street
London EC1M 6PU
Tel.: 020 7251 5860
Website: www.addaction.org.uk
One of the UK's largest specialist drug and alcohol treatment charities, it manages more than 120 services in 80 locations in England and Scotland. Working with families and loved ones forms a major part of Addaction's treatment ethos. The website gives details of the services offered to drug users and their families, and their location.

Adfam
25 Corsham Street
London N1 6DR
Tel.: 020 7553 7640 (NB – this is not a helpline)
Website: www.adfam.org.uk
An umbrella organization which campaigns for more support for families of drug addicts, Adfam provides an extensive range of publications targeted towards various specific groups who might be affected by a family

member's drug use, including grandparents, siblings and those living with bereavement. The website gives details of local support groups, a list of useful organizations, and supporting helplines for those affected by a family member's drug use.

After Adoption
Head Office
Unit 5, Citygate
5 Blantyre Street
Manchester M15 4JJ
Helpline: 0800 0 568 578
Website: www.afteradoption.co.uk
Works with children, families and adults and offers support throughout the adoption process.

The British Association for Counselling and Psychotherapy (BACP)
BACP House
15 St John's Business Park
Lutterworth LE17 4HB
General enquiries: 01455 883300
Website: www.bacp.co.uk
Information on finding a qualified therapist.

ChildLine
Helpline: 0800 1111
Website: www.childline.org.uk
A free and confidential helpline for children and young adults across the UK to talk about anything that worries them.

Children 1st (working name of the Royal Scottish Society for Prevention of Cruelty to Children)
83 Whitehouse Loan
Edinburgh EH9 1AT
Helpline: 0808 800 2222 (particularly for concerned parents)
Website: www.children1st.org.uk
Supports Scottish families under stress, protects children from harm and neglect, helps them to recover from abuse and promotes children's rights and interests.

Citizens Advice Bureau (Scotland)
Website: http://www.adviceguide.org.uk/scotland/your_family/family_and_personal_issues_index_scotland/kinship_care_scotland.htm
The website provides a simple guide for kinship carers in Scotland, including the law, legal terms and the benefits available to kinship carers. See also National Association of Kinship Carers.

Co-Dependents Anonymous
General enquiries: enquiries@coda-uk.org
Website: www.coda-uk.org

Families Anonymous
C/o Doddington & Rollo Community Association
Charlotte Despard Avenue
London SW11 5HD
Helpline: 0845 1200 660
Website: www.famanon.org.uk
A worldwide fellowship of relatives and friends of people involved in the abuse of mind-altering substances, or with related behavioural problems. It is a self-help organization with a programme based on the 12 Steps and 12 Traditions first formulated by Alcoholics Anonymous. Groups hold meetings regularly throughout the country, and any concerned person is encouraged to attend, even if there is only a suspicion of a problem.

Family Rights Group
Second Floor, The Print House
18 Ashwin Street
London E8 3DL
Tel.: 0808 801 0366 (free confidential help and advice service, 9.30 a.m. to 3.30 p.m., Monday to Friday)
Website: www.frg.org.uk
A charity in England and Wales which advises parents and other family members whose children are involved with or require children's social services because of welfare needs or concerns.

Grandparents Apart
Tel.: 0141 882 5658
Website: www.grandparentsapart.co.uk
A Scottish self-help network dedicated to easing the suffering of grandparents and grandchildren and extended families torn apart. The website gives details of other phone contacts.

Grandparents Association
Head Office, Moot House
The Stow
Harlow
Essex CM20 3AG
Helpline: 0845 434 9585
Website: www.grandparents-association.org.uk
A network of support groups around England and Wales offering confidential help and advice for grandparents bringing up their grandchildren, and

support for those who have lost contact with their grandchildren. It has a dedicated welfare benefits service.

Grandparents Plus
18 Victoria Park Square
London E2 9PF
Helpline: 0300 123 7015 (10 a.m. to 3 p.m., Monday to Friday)
Website: www.grandparents.plus.org.uk
A charity covering England and Wales which champions the vital role of grandparents and the wider family in children's lives, especially when they take on the caring role in difficult family circumstances.

Kinship Care Northern Ireland
Website: http://jacquelinewilliamson.wordpress.com/kinship-care-northern-ireland
Email: kinshipcare.ni@gmail.com
A charitable organization committed to helping and supporting grandparents and other family members who are caring for children of their extended families.

National Association of Kinship Carers
Website: http://kinshipcarers.me.uk
Led by and for kin carers, and covering England, Northern Ireland, Scotland and Wales, this association campaigns for better rights and entitlements for kinship carers and the children in their care. See also Citizens Advice Bureau (Scotland).

National Society for the Prevention of Cruelty to Children
Weston House
42 Curtain Road
London EC2A 3NH
Helpline: 0808 800 5000
Website: www.nspcc.org.uk
The helpline offers confidential advice if you are worried about a child's well-being. The website provides a useful list of warning signs that something may be wrong, plus parenting resources and advice on helping vulnerable children.

Parents Against Drug Abuse
12–14 Church Parade
Ellesmere Port CH65 2ER
Helpline: 08457 023867
Website: www.btinternet.com/~padahelp/
A national charity offering help and support to parents of drug users.

Scottish Families Affected by Drugs
Suite 2E, Ingram House
227 Ingram Street
Glasgow G1 1DA
Helpline: 08080 10 10 11
Website: www.sfad.org.uk
Supports families across Scotland who are affected by drug misuse, and raises awareness of the issues affecting them. It can direct you to services in your local area. The helpline is free and confidential, staffed by trained volunteers from 5 p.m. to 11 p.m., 7 days a week.

Women's Aid
Tel.: 0117 944 4411 (general enquiries)
Helpline: 0808 2000 247
Website: www.womensaid.org.uk
The key national charity working to end domestic violence against women and children, it supports a network of over 500 domestic and sexual violence services across the UK.

Resources on drugs, treatment and addiction, and related issues

The Alliance
32 Bloomsbury Street
London WC1B 3QJ
Helpline: 0845 122 8608
Website: www.m-alliance.org.uk
Provides advocacy, training and helpline services to those currently in drug or alcohol treatment, those who have accessed treatment in the past and those who may access treatment in the future.

Benzodiazepines
The website <www.benzo.org.uk/index/htm> contains a wealth of information on benzodiazepine addiction, withdrawal and recovery.

Black Poppy
Website: www.blackpoppy.org.uk
A health and lifestyle site aimed at drug users, which contains useful advice on health, and overdose management and prevention.

DrugScope
Prince Consort House
Suite 204, Second Floor

109–111 Farringdon Road
London EC1R 3BW
Tel.: 020 7520 7550
Website: www.drugscope.org.uk/resources/drugsearch
The UK's leading independent centre of expertise on drugs, and the national membership organization for the drug field. The website contains DrugSearch, an online encyclopaedia of drugs and their history, effects and the law relating to them.

FRANK
Helpline: 0800 77 66 00 (free and confidential, 24 hours a day, 365 days a year)
Website: www.talktofrank.com
The national drugs helpline, providing advice on all aspects of drugs and drug abuse in 120 languages, plus information on local services.

Narcotics Anonymous
Service Office
202 City Road
London EC1V 2PH
Tel.: 020 7251 4007 (general administrative enquiries, e.g. details of the 12-Step programme)
Helpline: 0300 999 1212
Website: www.ukna.org
A non-profit, non-religious fellowship or society of men and women for whom drugs have become a major problem. They are recovering addicts who meet regularly to help one another stay clean. There is a network of local meetings around the country. NA uses the 12-Step programme approach used by Alcoholics Anonymous. These steps include admitting to a drug problem; seeking help; self-appraisal; confidential self-disclosure; making amends where possible, where harm has been done; achieving a spiritual awakening and supporting other drug addicts who want to recover.

National Institute of Health and Clinical Excellence (NICE)
A booklet giving NICE guidelines on treatment for drug misuse (opiates and stimulants) for adults and young people aged 16 and over, whether patients or carers, may be downloaded from the following website: <www.nice.org.uk/nicemedia/live/11813/36009/36009.pdf>.

National Treatment Agency for Substance Misuse
Website: www.nta.nhs.uk
Part of the NHS, this agency was established in 2001 to improve the availability, capacity and effectiveness of drug treatment in England. Its publication *Getting Help for a Drug Problem: A guide to treatment* may be downloaded from the website. In 2008 the agency published *Supporting and Involving*

Carers, which may be downloaded from <www.adfam.org.uk/docs/supp-porting_and_involving_carers.pdf>.

Release
124–128 City Road
London EC1V 2NJ
Helpline: 0845 4500 215 (11 a.m. to 1 p.m./2 p.m. to 4 p.m., Monday to Friday)
Website: www.release.org.uk
The only specialist provider of legal services to drug users in the UK, resolving their housing, debt and welfare problems.

Re-Solv
30a High Street
Stone
Staffordshire ST15 8AW
Tel.: 01785 817885 (national information line)
Website: www.re-solv.org/
The national charity solely dedicated to the prevention of solvent and volatile-substance abuse.

St John Ambulance
27 St John's Lane
London EC1M 4BU
Tel.: 08700 10 49 50
Website: www.sja.org.uk
The UK's leading supplier of first-aid courses. The website contains useful information on chest compressions and resuscitation, and how to spot the first signs of an overdose.

Talking About Cannabis
Website: www.talkingaboutcannabis.com
A support and information website set up by the parent of a cannabis addict, and intended for anyone who has been affected by cannabis use.

UK Drug Rehab
Website: www.uk-rehab.com
A privately funded, non-profit-making project that aims to provide free, unbiased information on drug addiction, alcoholism, substance abuse, addiction treatment and drug rehab centres and clinics.

Further reading

The Road to Resilience. Washington, DC, American Psychological Association. A booklet that includes ways to build resilience, learning from your past, and resilience factors and strategies. Available at the following website: www.apa.org/helpcenter/road-resilience.aspx

Beattie, Melody, *Codependent No More: How to Stop Controlling Others and Start Caring for Yourself*. Center City, Minnesota, Hazelden Information and Education Services, 1989.
A useful insight into the concept of co-dependence.

Burton-Phillips, Elizabeth, *Mum Can You Lend Me Twenty Quid? What Drugs Did to My Family*. London, Piatkus, 2008.

Conyers, Beverly, *Everything Changes: Help for Families of Newly Recovering Addicts*. Center City, Minnesota, Hazelden, 2009.
Advice and support on helping a recovering addict.

Higgins, Gina O'Connell, *Resilient Adults: Overcoming a Cruel Past*. Oxford, Wiley, 1996.
A fascinating insight into the lives and strategies of adults who have overcome past trauma.

Johnson, Mark, *Wasted*. London, Sphere, 2008.
The story of a recovered heroin and crack addict, in his own words.

References

Studies and books

Ashton, H. (2002). *Benzodiazepines: How they work and how to withdraw* (a.k.a. The Ashton Manual). Published online at http://www.benzo.org.uk/manual/bzcha02.htm

Barber, J. G.and Crisp, B. R. (1995). 'The "pressures to change" approach to working with the partners of heavy drinkers'. *Addiction*, 90: 269–76.

Barnard, M. (2007). *Drug Addiction and Families*. London, Jessica Kingsley, p. 11.

Best, D. W., Ghufran, S., Day, E., Ray, R., Loaring, J. (2008). 'Breaking the habit: A retrospective analysis of desistance factors among formerly problematic heroin users'. *Drug Alcohol Review*, 27(6): 619–24.

Bloor, R. N., McAuley, R. and Smalldridge, N. (2005). 'Safe storage of methadone in the home – an audit of the effectiveness of safety information giving'. *Harm Reduction Journal*, 2: 9.

Bolton, J. M., Robinson, J., Sareen, J. (2009). 'Self-medication of mood disorders with alcohol and drugs in the National Epidemiological Survey on Alcohol and Related Conditions'. *Journal of Affective Disorders*, 115(3): 367–75.

Burton, L. (1992). 'Black grandparents rearing children of drug-addicted parents: Stressors, outcomes and social service needs'. *The Gerontologist*, 32(6): 744–51.

Chu, P. S., Kwok, S. C., Lam, K. M., Chu, T. Y., Chan, S. W., Man, C. W., Ma, W. K., Chui, K. L., Yiu, M. K., Chan, Y. C., Tse, M. L., Lau, F. L. (2007). ' "Street ketamine"-associated bladder dysfunction: A report of ten cases'. *Hong Kong Medical Journal*, 13: 311–13.

Conan Doyle, Sir Arthur. 'The Sign of Four'. *The Complete Sherlock Holmes*. London, Magpie Books, 1993, p. 89.

Copello, A., Templeton, L., Orford, J., Velleman, R. (2010). 'The 5-Step Method: Principles and practice'. *Drugs: Education, Prevention and Policy*, 17(s1): 86–99.

Copello, A., Templeton, L., Powell, J. (2009). *Adult family members and carers of dependent drug users: Prevalence, social cost, resource savings and treatment responses*. Report from the UK Drug Policy Commission.

Copello, A. G., Templeton, L., Velleman, R. (2006). 'Family interventions for drug and alcohol misuse: Is there a best practice?' *Current Opinion in Psychiatry*, 19(3): 271–6.

Dawson, D. A., Grant, B. F., Chou, S. P., Stinson, F. S. (2007). 'The impact of partner alcohol problems on women's physical and mental health'. *Journal of Studies on Alcohol and Drugs*, 68(1): 66–75.

Farrell, A. D. and White, K. S. (1998). 'Peer influences and drug use among urban adolescents: Family structure and parent-adolescent relationship as protective factors'. *Journal of Consulting and Clinical Psychology*, 66(2): 248–58.

Fernandez, A. C., Begley, E. A. and Marlatt, G. A. (2006). 'Family and peer interventions for adults: Past approaches and future directions'. *Psychology of Addictive Behaviors*, 20(2): 207–13.

Foltin, R. W., Fischman, M. W., Pedroso, J. J. and Pearlson, G. D. (1987). 'Marijuana and cocaine interactions in humans: Cardiovascular consequences'. *Pharmacology, Biochemistry and Behavior*, 28(4):459–64.

Gomberg, E. L. (1989). 'On terms used and abused: The concept of "codependency"'. *Drugs and Society*, 3: 113–32.

Gorman, J.M. and Rooney, J. F. (1979). 'The influence of Al-Anon on the coping behavior of wives of alcoholics'. *Journal of Studies on Alcohol*, 40: 1030–8.

Hurcom, C., Copello, A. and Orford, J. (2000). 'The family and alcohol: Effects of excessive drinking and conceptualizations of spouses over recent decades'. *Substance Use and Misuse*, 35(4): 473–502.

Ives, R. and Ghelani, P. (2006). 'Polydrug use (the use of drugs in combination): A brief review'. *Drugs: Education, Prevention and Policy*, 13(3): 225–32.

Kingston, A., Morgan, A., Jorm, A. F., Hall, K., Hart, L. M., Kelly, C. M., Lubman, D. I. (2011). 'Helping someone with problem drug use: A Delphi consensus study of consumers, carers, and clinicians'. *BMC Psychiatry*, 11: 3 (5 January).

Leeies, M., Paguras, J., Sareen, J., Bolton, J. M. (2010). 'The use of alcohol and drugs to self-medicate symptoms of posttraumatic stress disorder'. *Depression and Anxiety*, 27(8): 731–6.

Leri, F., Bruneau, J. and Stewart, J. (2003). 'Understanding polydrug use: Review of heroin and cocaine co-use'. *Addiction*, 98(1): 7–22.

Liepman, M. R., Nirenberg, T. D. and Begin, A. M. (1989). 'Evaluation of a program designed to help family and significant others to motivate resistant alcoholics into recovery'. *American Journal of Alcohol and Drug Abuse*, 15(2): 209–21.

Loneck, B., Garrett, J. A. and Banks, M. (1996). 'The Johnson Intervention and relapse during outpatient treatment'. *American Journal of Alcohol and Drug Abuse*, 22(3): 363–75.

Macdonald, D., Russell, P., Bland, N., Morrison, A. and De la Cruz, C. (2002). 'Supporting families and carers of drug users: A review'. Centre for Research on Families and Relationships at the University of Edinburgh, published by the Effective Interventions Unit, Scotland.

Marlowe, D. B., Merikle, E. P., Kirby, K. C., Festinger, D. S., McLellan, A. T. (2001). 'Multidimensional assessment of perceived treatment-entry pressures among substance abusers'. *Psychology of Addictive Behaviors*, 15(2): 97–108.

Mental Health First Aid Training and Research Program, *Helping Someone*

With Problem Drug Use: Mental health first aid guidelines. Melbourne: Orygen Youth Health Research Centre, University of Melbourne, 2009. May be downloaded from <http://www.mhfa.com.au>.

Meyers, R., Miller, W., Hill, D. and Tonigan, J. (1998), Community Reinforcement and Family Training (CRAFT). 'Engaging unmotivated drug users in treatment'. *Journal of Substance Abuse*, 10(3): 291–308.

National Treatment Agency for Substance Misuse (2008). *Getting Help for a Drug Problem: A guide to treatment*.

National Treatment Agency for Substance Misuse (2008). *Supporting and Involving Carers*. May be downloaded from <http://www.adfam.org.uk/docs/supporting_and_involving_carers.pdf>.

Nutt, D., King, L. A., Saulsbury, W. and Blakemore, C. (2007). 'Development of a rational scale to assess the harm of drugs of potential misuse'. *Lancet*, 369(9566): 1047–53.

Orford, J. (2010). 'Commentary on Roozen et al (2010): Involving families in addiction treatment – the way forward'. *Addiction*, 105(10): 1739–40.

Orford, J., Copello, A., Velleman, R. and Templeton, L. (2010). Family members affected by a close relative's addiction: The stress-strain-coping-support model'. *Drugs: Education, Prevention and Policy*, 17(s1): 36–43.

Orford, J., Natera, G., Davies, J., Nava, A., Mora, J., Rigby, K., Bradbury, C., Bowie, N., Copello, A. and Velleman, R. (1998). 'Tolerate, engage or withdraw: A study of the structure of families coping with alcohol and drug problems in South West England and Mexico City'. *Addiction*, 93(12): 1799–1813.

Orford, J., Templeton, L., Velleman, R. and Copello, A. (2005). 'Family members of relatives with alcohol, drug and gambling problems: A set of standardized questionnaires for assessing stress, coping and strain'. *Addiction*, 100(11): 1611–24.

Orford, J., Velleman, R., Copello, A., Templeton, L. and Ibanga, A. (2010). 'The experiences of affected family members: A summary of two decades of qualitative research'. *Drugs: Education, Prevention and Policy*, 17(s1): 44–62.

Parker, H., Williams, L. and Aldridge, J. (2002). 'The normalization of "sensible" recreational drug use: Further evidence from the North West England Longitudinal Study'. *Sociology*, 36: 941–64.

Pilkington, H. (2007). 'Beyond "peer pressure": rethinking drug use and "youth culture"'. *International Journal of Drug Policy*, 18(3): 213–24.

Prochaska, J. and DiClemente, C. (1983). 'Stages and processes of self-change of smoking: towards an integrative model of change'. *Journal of Consulting and Clinical Psychology*, 51(3): 390–5.

Reuter, R. and Stevens, A. (2007). *An Analysis of UK Drug Policy*. London: UK Drug Policy Commission report.

Roozen, H. G., de Waart, R. and van der Kroft, P. (2010). 'Community reinforcement and family training: An effective option to engage treatment-resistant substance-abusing individuals in treatment'. *Addiction*, 105(10): 1729–38.

Stanton, M. D. (2004). 'Getting reluctant substance abusers to engage in treatment/self-help: A review of outcomes and clinical options'. *Journal of Marital and Family Therapy*, 30(2): 165–82.

Velleman, R., Bennett, G., Miller, T., Orford, J., Rigby, K. and Tod, A. (1993). 'The families of problem drug users: A study of 50 close relatives'. *Addiction*, 88: 1281–9.

Velleman, R. and Templeton, L. (2007). 'Understanding and modifying the impact of parents' substance misuse on children'. *Advances in Psychiatric Treatment*, 13: 79–89.

Volkow, N. D. (2005). 'What do we know about drug addiction?' *American Journal of Psychiatry*, 162(8): 1401–2.

White, W. (2000). 'Addiction as a disease: The birth of a concept'. *Counselor*, 1(1): 46–51, 73.

Media references

'One in 50 admit to drug addiction', Jamie Doward, *The Guardian* (Society section), 26 July 2009.

'Ketamine link to bladder failure', BBC News, 4 February 2009. <http://news.bbc.co.uk/1/hi/england/bristol/7867449.stm>

'Six out of 10 male drug addicts abuse their partners, Spanish study finds', *ScienceDaily*, 3 March 2011.

'Drink and drugs push grandparents into caring roles' (<http://www.nurseryworld.co.uk/news/1053165/Drink-drugs-push-grandparents-caring-roles>).

Web references

DSM proposed revisions

http://www.dsm5.org/ProposedRevisions/Pages/proposedrevision.aspx?rid=431#

GHB (gamma-hydroxybutyrate)

http://www.national.slam.nhs.uk/about-us/media/mediareleases/partydrug
dependencehighergaymen/

http://www.erowid.org/chemicals/ghb/ghb.shtml

GBL (gamma-butyrolactone)

http://menmedia.co.uk/manchestereveningnews/news/s/1138919_
pictured_girl_ravaged_by_party_drug_gbl

Most addictive drugs
http://www.druglibrary.org/Schaffer/library/basicfax5.htm

Risks of injecting and HIV/hepatitis C statistics
http://www.nhs.uk/Conditions/Drug-misuse/Pages/Introduction.aspx

Transform Drug Policy Foundation
http://www.tdpf.org.uk/Policy_Timeline.htm
A charitable think tank that seeks to draw public attention to the fact that the prohibition of drugs is itself the major cause of drug-related harm, and that it should be replaced by effective, just and humane government control and regulation. The website refers to their guide to the history of drug prohibition laws.

World Health Organization International Classification of Diseases and Related Health Problems
http://apps.who.int/classifications/apps/icd/icd10online/

Index